&Medicare You

2015

2015

This is the official U.S. government Medicare handbook.

★ What's important in 2015 (page 12)
★ What Medicare covers (page 35)

DEPARTMENT OF HEALTH & HUMAN SERVICES · USA

CENTERS FOR MEDICARE & MEDICAID SERVICES

Want to read this information online?

Sign up at Medicare.gov/gopaperless to get your future "Medicare & You" information electronically (also called the "eHandbook"). We'll send you an email next September when the new eHandbook is available. The online version of the handbook contains all the same information you get in the printed version. Even better, the information on the web is updated regularly, so you can instantly find the most up-to-date Medicare information. You won't get a printed copy of your handbook in the mail if you choose to get it electronically.

Have an eReader (like an iPad, NOOK, Sony Reader, or Kindle)?

Visit Medicare.gov/publications to download a free digital version of this handbook to your eReader. This option is

available for all eReader devices. You can get the same important information that's included in the printed version in an easy-to-read format that you can take anywhere you go. You'll still get a printed copy of the handbook in the mail if you choose to download the digital version.

Please keep this handbook for future reference.
The information in this booklet describes the Medicare program at the time this booklet was printed. Changes may occur after printing. Visit Medicare.gov, or call 1-800-MEDICARE (1-800-633-4227) to get the most current information. TTY users should call 1-877-486-2048.

"Medicare & You" isn't a legal document. Official Medicare Program legal guidance is contained in the relevant statutes, regulations, and rulings.

Welcome to "Medicare & You" 2015

Our nation's health care system has gone through a historic transformation. More Americans have the peace of mind that comes from health coverage, and your Medicare program continues to grow stronger and provide important benefits to keep you healthy.

Let's take a look at some of those benefits—so you can get the most out of this year's handbook and your Medicare coverage:

- Covered preventive services—Millions of people with Medicare have taken advantage of expanded benefits like preventive services, cancer screenings, and yearly "Wellness" visits—without paying a dollar out-of-pocket. You can use the checklist on page 61 to help you track the preventive services you had and understand the services you might need.

- Continued savings in the Part D coverage gap—You can join the millions of people with Medicare who have already saved money on covered drugs. In 2015, if you enter the coverage gap, you'll pay 45% of the plan's cost for covered brand-name drugs and 65% of the cost for covered generic drugs. See pages 101–102 to learn more.

- Choice of plans in your area—You have a choice of how you get your Medicare coverage. Did you know that Medicare.gov/find-a-plan has a list of the Medicare health and prescription drug plans that are offered in your area? This list includes premiums, out-of-pocket costs, plan ratings, and more to help you get started finding a plan that meets your individual needs.

As always, if you have specific questions about Medicare, visit Medicare.gov to find the answers you need. You also can call 1-800-MEDICARE (1-800-633-4227). TTY users should call 1-877-486-2048.

Yours in good health,

/s/

/s/

Sylvia M. Burwell

Marilyn B. Tavenner

Secretary

Administrator

U.S. Department of Health and Human Services

Centers for Medicare & Medicaid Services

Contents

Index Find a Specific Topic

Note: The page numbers shown in **bold** provide the most detailed information.

> **Note:** The page numbers shown in **bold** provide the most detailed information.

Note: The page numbers shown in **bold** provide the most detailed information.

Note: The page numbers shown in **bold** provide the most detailed information.

Note: The page numbers shown in **bold** provide the most detailed information.

What's Important in 2015

Stay healthy with Medicare-covered preventive services

Medicare pays for many preventive services that can help prevent illness or detect health problems early when they're easier to treat. Ask your health care provider what services you need.

See page 61.

Keep track of your personal health information

Medicare has expanded its Blue Button to provide better access to your Medicare claims and personal health information.

See page 136.

Continue to get help in the prescription drug coverage gap

If you reach the coverage gap in your Medicare prescription drug coverage, you'll qualify for some savings on brand-name and generic drugs.

See page 101–102.

Find out what you pay for Medicare (Part A and Part B)

The 2015 Medicare premium and deductible amounts weren't available at the time of printing. To get the most up-to-date cost information, visit Medicare.gov or call 1-800-MEDICARE (1-800-633-4227). TTY users should call 1-877-486-2048.

Important Enrollment Information

You don't need to sign up for Medicare each year. However, each year you'll have a chance to review your coverage and make changes.

Coverage and costs change yearly

Definitions of blue words are on pages 145–148.

Medicare health and drug plans can make changes each year—things like cost, coverage, and which providers and pharmacies are in their networks. If you're in a Medicare health or prescription drug plan, always review the materials your plan sends you, like the "Evidence of Coverage" (EOC) and "Annual Notice of Change" (ANOC). Make sure your plan will still meet your needs for the following year. If you're satisfied that your current plan will meet your needs for next year and it's still being offered, you don't need to do anything.

Open Enrollment Period

Mark your calendar with these important dates! In most cases, this may be the only chance you have each year to make a change to your health and prescription drug coverage.

October 1, 2014	**Start comparing your coverage with other options.** You may be able to save money by comparing all of your options. See page 18 for information on comparing plans.
October 15– December 7, 2014	**Change your Medicare health or prescription drug coverage for 2015, if you decide to.** See pages 86–87 and 98–99 for other times you may be able to switch your coverage.
January 1, 2015	**New coverage begins if you make a change during Open Enrollment.** New costs and benefit changes also begin if you keep your existing Medicare health or prescription drug coverage, and your plan makes changes.

Notes

Section 1—
Learn How Medicare Works

Medicare is health insurance for people 65 or older, people under 65 with certain disabilities, and people of any age with End-Stage Renal Disease (ESRD) (permanent kidney failure requiring dialysis or a kidney transplant).

What are the different parts of Medicare?

Medicare Part A (Hospital Insurance) helps cover:

See pages 35–39.

- Inpatient care in hospitals
- Skilled nursing facility care
- Hospice care
- Home health care

Medicare Part B (Medical Insurance) helps cover:

See pages 40–60.

- Services from doctors and other health care providers
- Outpatient care
- Home health care
- Durable medical equipment
- Some preventive services

Medicare Part C (Medicare Advantage):

See pages 75–90.

- Includes all benefits and services covered under Part A and Part B
- Usually includes Medicare prescription drug coverage (Part D) as part of the plan
- Run by Medicare-approved private insurance companies
- May include extra benefits and services for an extra cost

Medicare Part D (Medicare prescription drug coverage):

See pages 97–110.

- Helps cover the cost of prescription drugs
- Run by Medicare-approved private insurance companies
- May help lower your prescription drug costs and help protect against higher costs in the future

How can I get my Medicare coverage?

You can choose different ways to get your Medicare coverage:

1. You can choose **Original Medicare**. If you want prescription drug coverage, you must join a Medicare Prescription Drug Plan (Part D). If you don't join a Medicare drug plan when you're first eligible, and you don't have other creditable prescription drug coverage (for example, from an employer or union), **you may pay a late enrollment penalty if you choose to join later**. See pages 104–105 for more information about the late enrollment penalty.

2. You can choose to join a **Medicare Advantage Plan (like an HMO or PPO)** if one's available in your area. The Medicare Advantage Plan may include Medicare prescription drug coverage. In most cases, you must take the drug coverage that comes with the Medicare health plan if it's offered. In some types of plans that don't offer drug coverage, you may be able to join a Medicare Prescription Drug Plan.

If you don't join a Medicare Advantage Plan, you'll have Original Medicare. See the next page for more information about your coverage choices and the decisions you need to make.

This handbook has basic information. You'll need more detailed information than this handbook provides to make an informed choice. Before making any decisions, learn as much as you can about the types of coverage available to you. See pages 18 and 20 to find out how to get personalized help.

Definitions of blue words are on pages 145–148.

What are my Medicare coverage choices?

There are 2 main choices for how you get your Medicare coverage. Use these steps to help you decide.

Step 1

Decide if you want Original Medicare or a Medicare Advantage Plan.

Original Medicare includes
Part A (Hospital Insurance) and/or Part B (Medical Insurance)

- Medicare provides this coverage directly.
- You have your choice of doctors, hospitals, and other providers that accept Medicare.
- Generally, you or your supplemental coverage pay deductibles and coinsurance.
- You usually pay a monthly premium for Part B.

See pages 67–73.

Step 2

Decide if you want prescription drug coverage (Part D).

- If you want drug coverage, **you must join a Medicare Prescription Drug Plan.** You usually pay a monthly premium.
- These plans are run by private companies approved by Medicare.

See pages 97–110.

Step 3

Decide if you want supplemental coverage.

- You may want to get coverage that fills gaps in Original Medicare coverage. You can choose to buy a Medicare Supplement Insurance (Medigap) policy from a private company.
- Costs vary by policy and company.
- Employers/unions may offer similar coverage.

See pages 91–96.

Medicare Advantage Plan
(like an HMO or PPO)

Part C includes BOTH Part A (Hospital Insurance) and Part B (Medical Insurance)

- Private insurance companies approved by Medicare provide this coverage.
- In most plans, you need to use plan doctors, hospitals, and other providers or you may pay more or all of the costs.
- You may pay a monthly premium (in addition to your Part B premium) and a copayment or coinsurance for covered services.
- Costs, extra coverage, and rules vary by plan.

See pages 75–90.

Step 2

Decide if you want Medicare prescription drug coverage (Part D).

- If you want drug coverage, and it's offered by your Medicare Advantage Plan, **in most cases, you must get it through your plan.**
- In some types of plans that don't offer drug coverage, you can join a Medicare Prescription Drug Plan.

See page 78.

Note: If you join a Medicare Advantage Plan, you can't use Medicare Supplement Insurance (Medigap) to pay for out-of-pocket costs you have in the Medicare Advantage Plan. If you already have a Medicare Advantage Plan, you can't be sold a Medigap policy. You can only use a Medigap policy if you disenroll from your Medicare Advantage Plan and return to Original Medicare. See page 95.

In addition to the options listed above, you may be able to join other types of Medicare health plans. See pages 88–89. Some people may have other coverage like employer or union, Medicaid, military, or veterans' benefits. See pages 108–110.

What if I need help deciding how to get my Medicare?

1. **Visit the Medicare Plan Finder at Medicare.gov/find-a-plan.**
   The Medicare Plan Finder lets you compare plans by plan type and
   find out what the coverage, benefits, and estimated costs would be in
   each plan. It also shows you how Medicare has rated the plans' quality
   and performance. You can use the Medicare Plan Finder to enroll in a
   Medicare plan. Here's an example of what you may see:

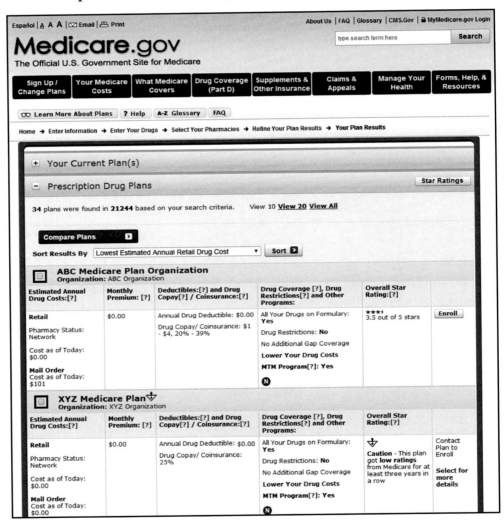

Definitions
of blue words
are on pages
145–148.

2. **Get personalized counseling about choosing coverage.** See pages
   141–144 for the phone number of your State Health Insurance
   Assistance Program (SHIP).

3. **Call 1-800-MEDICARE (1-800-633-4227) and say "Agent."** TTY
   users should call 1-877-486-2048. If you need help in a language other
   than English or Spanish, let the customer service representative know.

What should I consider when choosing or changing my coverage?

Convenience	Where are the doctors' offices? What are their hours? Do the doctors use electronic health records or prescribe electronically? Which pharmacies can you use? Is the pharmacy you use in the plan's network? If it's in the network and your plan has preferred pharmacies, is your pharmacy preferred? (You may pay more at non-preferred pharmacies.) Can you get your prescriptions by mail?
Cost	How much are your premiums, deductibles, and other costs? How much do you pay for services like hospital stays or doctor visits? Is there a yearly limit on what you pay out-of-pocket? Your costs may vary and may be different if you don't follow the coverage rules.
Coverage	How well does the plan cover the services you need?
Doctor and hospital choice	Do your doctors and other health care providers accept the type of coverage you have? Are the doctors you want to see accepting new patients? Do you have to choose your hospital and health care providers from a network? Do you need to get referrals?
Prescription drugs	Do you need to join a Medicare drug plan? Are your drugs covered under the plan's formulary? Are there any coverage rules that apply to your prescriptions?
Quality of care	Are you satisfied with your medical care? The quality of care and services offered by plans and other health care providers can vary. Medicare has information to help you compare how well plans and providers work to give you the best care possible. See pages 136–137.
Travel	Will you have coverage in another state or outside the U.S.?
Your other coverage	Do you have, or are you eligible for, other types of health or prescription drug coverage (like from a former or current employer or union)? If so, read the materials from your insurer or plan, or call them to find out how the coverage works with, or is affected by, Medicare. If you have coverage through a former or current employer or union or other source, talk to your benefits administrator, insurer, or plan before making any changes to your coverage. If you drop your coverage, you may not be able to get it back.

Where can I get my questions answered?

1-800-MEDICARE (1-800-633-4227)

Get general or claims-specific Medicare information, request documents in alternate formats, and make changes to your Medicare coverage. If you need help in a language other than English or Spanish, say "Agent" to talk to a customer service representative.

TTY 1-877-486-2048
Medicare.gov

Benefits Coordination & Recovery Center (BCRC)

Find out if Medicare or your other insurance pays first. Let the BCRC know if you have other insurance, or if you need to report changes in your insurance information.

1-855-798-2627
TTY 1-855-797-2627

Department of Defense

Get information about TRICARE for Life and the TRICARE Pharmacy Program.

1-866-773-0404 (TFL)
TTY 1-866-773-0405
1-877-363-1303 (Pharmacy)
TTY 1-877-540-6261
tricare.mil/mybenefit

Department of Health and Human Services Office for Civil Rights

Contact if you think you were discriminated against or if your health information privacy rights were violated.

1-800-368-1019
TTY 1-800-537-7697
hhs.gov/ocr

Definitions of blue words are on pages 145–148.

Department of Veterans Affairs

Contact if you're a veteran or have served in the U.S. military and you have questions about VA benefits.

1-800-827-1000
TTY 1-800-829-4833
va.gov

Office of Personnel Management

Get information about the Federal Employee Health Benefits (FEHB) Program for current and retired federal employees.

Retirees: 1-888-767-6738
TTY 1-800-878-5707
opm.gov/healthcare-insurance

Active federal employees: Contact your Benefits Officer. Visit apps.opm.gov/abo for a list of Benefits Officers.

Quality Improvement Organization (QIO)

Ask questions or report complaints about the quality of care for a Medicare-covered service you got, or if you think Medicare coverage for your service is ending too soon (for example, if your hospital says that you must be discharged and you disagree.)

We've made some changes to the QIO program to make sure your needs are better met. We've created a specific QIO just to address the concerns of people with Medicare and their families. These QIOs are called Beneficiary and Family Centered Care QIOs. There will be a second QIO that will work with hospitals and doctors to help them with quality improvement. These QIOs will be called Quality Innovation Network QIOs.

Visit qioprogram.org to get more information. Visit Medicare.gov/contacts, or call 1-800-MEDICARE to get the phone number of your QIO.

Railroad Retirement Board (RRB)

If you have benefits from the RRB, call them to change your address or name, check eligibility, enroll in Medicare, replace your Medicare card, or report a death.

1-877-772-5772
TTY 1-312-751-4701
rrb.gov

Social Security

Get a replacement Medicare or Social Security card, report a change to your address or name, find out if you're eligible for Part A and/or Part B and how to enroll, apply for Extra Help with Medicare prescription drug costs, ask questions about Part A and Part B premiums, and report a death.

1-800-772-1213
TTY 1-800-325-0778
socialsecurity.gov

State Health Insurance Assistance Program (SHIP)

Get personalized Medicare counseling at no cost to you.
See pages 141–144 for the phone number.

Definitions of blue words are on pages 145–148.

Section 2—

Signing Up for Medicare Part A & Part B

Some people get Part A and Part B automatically

If you're already getting benefits from Social Security or the Railroad Retirement Board (RRB), you'll automatically get Part A and Part B starting the first day of the month you turn 65. (If your birthday is on the first day of the month, Part A and Part B will start the first day of the prior month.)

If you're under 65 and disabled, you'll automatically get Part A and Part B after you get disability benefits from Social Security for 24 months or certain disability benefits from the RRB for 24 months.

If you have ALS (Amyotrophic Lateral Sclerosis, also called Lou Gehrig's disease), you'll get Part A and Part B automatically the month your disability benefits begin.

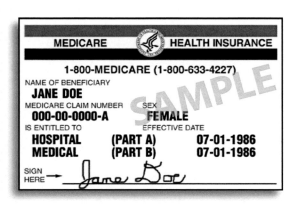

If you're automatically enrolled, you'll get your red, white, and blue Medicare card in the mail 3 months before your 65th birthday or 25th month of disability benefits. If you're going to wait to get Part B, follow the instructions that come with the card, and send the card back. If you keep the card, you keep Part B and will pay Part B premiums. See pages 26–27 for help deciding if you should wait to get Part B.

Note: If you don't get your card in the mail, call Social Security at 1-800-772-1213 and make sure they have the correct address on file. TTY users should call 1-800-325-0778.

Some people have to sign up for Part A and/or Part B

If you're close to 65, but not getting Social Security or Railroad Retirement Board (RRB) benefits and you want Part A and Part B, you'll need to sign up. Contact Social Security 3 months before you turn 65. You can also apply for Part A and Part B at socialsecurity.gov/retirement. If you worked for a railroad, contact the RRB.

If you have End-Stage Renal Disease (ESRD), you'll need to sign up. Contact Social Security to find out when and how to sign up for Part A

and Part B. For more information, visit Medicare.gov/publications to view the booklet "Medicare Coverage of Kidney Dialysis & Kidney Transplant Services." You can also call 1-800-MEDICARE (1-800-633-4227) to find out if a copy can be mailed to you. TTY users should call 1-877-486-2048.

Important! **If you live in Puerto Rico and get benefits from Social Security or the RRB,** you'll automatically get Part A the first day of the month you turn 65 or after you get disability benefits for 24 months. **However, if you want Part B, you'll need to sign up for it. If you don't sign up for Part B when you're first eligible, you may have to pay a late enrollment penalty for as long as you have Part B.** See page 25. Contact our local Social Security office or RRB for more information.

Note: To get Part A and/or Part B, you must be a U.S. citizen or lawfully present in the U.S.

Where can I get more information?

Call Social Security at 1-800-772-1213 for more information about your Medicare eligibility and to sign up for Part A and/or Part B. TTY users should call 1-800-325-0778. If you worked for a railroad or get RRB benefits, call the RRB at 1-877-772-5772. TTY users should call 1-312-751-4701.

You can also get personalized health insurance counseling at no cost to you from your State Health Insurance Assistance Program (SHIP). See pages 141–144 for the phone number.

If I'm not automatically enrolled, when can I sign up?

If you want Part A and/or Part B, you can sign up during the times listed below. **In most cases, if you don't sign up for Medicare when you're first eligible, you may have to pay a late enrollment penalty for as long as you have Part B.**

Initial Enrollment Period

You can sign up for Part A and/or Part B during the 7-month period that begins 3 months before the month you turn 65, includes the month you turn 65, and ends 3 months after the month you turn 65.

If you sign up for Part A and/or Part B during the first 3 months of your Initial Enrollment Period, in most cases, your coverage starts the first day of your birthday month. However, if your birthday is on the first day of the month, your coverage will start the first day of the prior month.

If you enroll in Part A and/or Part B the month you turn 65 or during the last 3 months of your Initial Enrollment Period, the start date for your Medicare coverage will be delayed.

General Enrollment Period

If you didn't sign up for Part A and/or Part B (for which you must pay premiums) during your Initial Enrollment Period and you aren't eligible for a Special Enrollment Period (see below), you can sign up between January 1–March 31 each year. Your coverage will begin July 1 of that year. **You may have to pay a higher Part A and/or Part B premium for late enrollment.** See pages 32 and 33.

Special Enrollment Period

Once your Initial Enrollment Period ends, you may have the chance to sign up for Medicare during a Special Enrollment Period. If you didn't sign up for Part A and/or Part B when you were first eligible because you're covered under a group health plan based on current employment (your own, a spouse's, or if you're disabled, a family member's), you can sign up for Part A and/or Part B:

- Anytime you're still covered by the group health plan
- During the 8-month period that begins the month after the employment ends or the coverage ends, whichever happens first

---

Remember, if you live in Puerto Rico, you don't automatically get Part B. You must call Social Security at 1-800-772-1213 to sign up for it. TTY users should call 1-800-325-0778.

Definitions of blue words are on pages 145–148.

Usually, you don't pay a late enrollment penalty if you sign up during a Special Enrollment Period. This Special Enrollment Period doesn't apply to people with End-Stage Renal Disease (ESRD). See page 24. You may also qualify for a Special Enrollment Period if you're a volunteer serving in a foreign country.

Important!

COBRA (Consolidated Omnibus Budget Reconciliation Act) coverage and retiree health plans aren't considered coverage based on current employment. You're not eligible for a Special Enrollment Period when that coverage ends. To avoid paying a higher premium, make sure you sign up for Medicare when you're first eligible. See page 109 for more information about COBRA coverage.

To learn more about enrollment periods, visit Medicare.gov/publications to view the booklet "Enrolling in Medicare Part A & Part B." You can also call 1-800-MEDICARE (1-800-633-4227) to find out if a copy can be mailed to you. TTY users should call 1-877-486-2048.

Should I get Part B?

This information can help you decide:

Employer or union coverage—If you or your spouse (or family member if you're disabled) is still working and you have health coverage through that employer or union, contact your employer or union benefits administrator to find out how your coverage works with Medicare. This includes federal or state employment, and active duty military service. It may be to your advantage to delay Part B enrollment. You can sign up for Part B without paying a penalty any time you have health coverage based on your (or your spouse's) current employment. COBRA and retiree health coverage don't count as current employer coverage. See page 28 to find out how your other insurance will work with Medicare.

Once the employment or coverage based on current employment ends (whichever happens first), 3 things happen:

Definitions of blue words are on pages 145–148.

1. You have 8 months to sign up for Part B without a penalty. **This period will run whether or not you choose COBRA. If you choose COBRA, don't wait until your COBRA ends to enroll in Part B.** If you don't enroll in Part B during the 8 months after the employment ends, you may have to pay a penalty after you enroll for as long as you have Part B. You won't be able to enroll until the next General Enrollment Period, and you'll have to wait until July 1 of that year before your coverage begins. This may cause a gap in your health care coverage.

2. You may be able to get COBRA coverage, which continues your health insurance through the employer's plan (in most cases for only 18 months) but probably at a higher cost to you.

   ▪ If you already have COBRA coverage when you enroll in Medicare, your COBRA will probably end.

   ▪ If you become eligible for COBRA coverage after you're already enrolled in Medicare, you must be allowed to take the COBRA coverage. If you choose COBRA, it will always be secondary to Medicare, unless you have End-Stage Renal Disease (ESRD).

3. When you sign up for Part B, your Medigap Open Enrollment Period begins. See page 94.

TRICARE—If you have TRICARE (insurance for active-duty military, military retirees, and their families), **you must enroll in Part A and Part B when you're first eligible to keep your TRICARE coverage.** However, if you're an active-duty service member, or the spouse or dependent child of an active-duty service member:

▪ You don't have to enroll in Part B to keep your TRICARE coverage while the service member is on active duty.

▪ Before the active-duty service member retires, you must enroll in Part B to keep TRICARE without a break in coverage.

▪ You can get Part B during a Special Enrollment Period if you have Medicare because you're 65 or older, or you're disabled.

▪ You should enroll in Part A and Part B when you're first eligible based on ESRD.

▪ After the active-duty service member retires, the TRICARE coverage becomes TRICARE for Life (TFL), which acts as a supplement to Medicare.

▪ Medicare pays first for Medicare-covered services. TRICARE will pay the Medicare deductible and coinsurance amounts and for any service TRICARE covers that Medicare doesn't cover. You pay the costs of services Medicare or TRICARE doesn't cover.

How does my other insurance work with Medicare?

When you have other insurance (like employer group health coverage), there are rules that decide whether Medicare or your other insurance pays first. Use this chart to see who pays first.

If you have **retiree** insurance (insurance from your or your spouse's former employment)...	Medicare pays first.
If you're 65 or older, have group health plan coverage based on your or your spouse's **current** employment, and the employer has **20 or more employees**...	Your group health plan pays first.
If you're 65 or older, have group health plan coverage based on your or your spouse's **current** employment, and the employer has **less than 20 employees**...	Medicare pays first.
If you're under 65 and disabled, have group health plan coverage based on your or a family member's **current** employment, and the employer has **100 or more employees**...	Your group health plan pays first.
If you're under 65 and disabled, have group health plan coverage based on your or a family member's **current** employment, and the employer has **less than 100 employees**...	Medicare pays first.
If you have Medicare because of End-Stage Renal Disease (ESRD)...	Your group health plan will pay first for the first 30 months after you become eligible to enroll in Medicare. Medicare will pay first after this 30-month period.

Definitions of blue words are on pages 145–148.

Note: In some cases, your employer may join with other employers or unions to form a multiple-employer plan. If this happens, the size of the largest employer/union determines whether Medicare pays first or second.

Here are some important facts to remember:

- The insurance that pays first (primary payer) pays up to the limits of its coverage.
- The insurance that pays second (secondary payer) only pays if there are costs the primary insurer didn't cover.
- The secondary payer (which may be Medicare) might not pay all of the uncovered costs.
- If your employer insurance is the secondary payer, you might need to enroll in Part B before your insurance will pay.

Medicare might pay second if you're in an accident or have a workers' compensation case in which other insurance covers your injury and is paying first. In these situations, you or your lawyer should tell Medicare as soon as possible. These types of insurance usually pay first:

- No-fault insurance (including automobile insurance)
- Liability insurance (including automobile and self-insurance)
- Black lung benefits
- Workers' compensation

Note: Medicare may pay conditionally if the no-fault, liability, or workers' compensation insurance hasn't settled on the claim. If Medicare makes a conditional payment for an item or service, and you get a settlement, judgment, award, or other payment for that item or service from an insurance company later, the conditional payment must be repaid to Medicare. You're responsible for making sure Medicare gets repaid for the conditional payment.

Medicaid never pays first for services that Medicare covers.
Medicaid will only pay after Medicare, employer group health plans, and/or Medicare Supplement Insurance (Medigap) policies have paid.

For more information, visit Medicare.gov/publications to view the booklet "Medicare & Other Health Benefits: Your Guide to Who Pays First." You can also call 1-800-MEDICARE (1-800-633-4227) to find out if a copy can be mailed to you. TTY users should call 1-877-486-2048.

Important!

If you have other insurance, be sure to tell your health care provider, hospital, and pharmacy. If you have questions about who pays first, or you need to update your other insurance information, call Medicare's Benefits Coordination & Recovery Center (BCRC) at 1-855-798-2627. TTY users should call 1-855-797-2627. You also can contact your employer or union benefits administrator. You may need to give your Medicare number to your other insurers so your bills are paid correctly and on time.

Medicare and the Health Insurance Marketplace

The Health Insurance Marketplace, a key part of the Affordable Care Act, is a way for qualified individuals, families, and qualified employees of small businesses to get health coverage. Medicare isn't part of the Marketplace.

If I have Medicare, do I need to do anything?

As long as you have Medicare Part A coverage, you're considered covered and you don't have to get any additional coverage.

If you **only** have Medicare Part B, you aren't considered to have minimum essential coverage. This means you may have to pay a fee for not having coverage.

Can I get a Marketplace plan instead of Medicare, or can I get a Marketplace plan in addition to Medicare?

Generally, no. **It's against the law for someone who knows you have Medicare to sell you a Marketplace plan, because that would duplicate your coverage.**

However, if you're employed and your employer offers employer-based coverage through the Marketplace, you may be eligible to get that type of coverage.

Note: The Marketplace doesn't offer Medicare Supplement Insurance (Medigap) policies, Medicare Advantage Plans, or Medicare drug plans (Part D).

Definitions of blue words are on pages 145–148.

What if I become eligible for Medicare after I join a Marketplace plan?

You can get a Marketplace plan to cover you before your Medicare coverage begins. You can cancel the Marketplace plan when your Medicare coverage starts. When you're eligible for Medicare, you'll have an Initial Enrollment Period to sign up (see page 25). In most cases it's to your advantage to sign up when you're first eligible because:

- When you're considered eligible for Medicare Part A, you won't qualify for Marketplace tax credits to help pay your premiums or reductions in cost-sharing that may be available through the Marketplace.

- If you enroll in Medicare after your Initial Enrollment Period ends, you may have to pay a late enrollment penalty for as long as you have Medicare.

Note: You can keep your Marketplace plan after your Medicare coverage starts. However, once your Part A coverage starts, any premium tax credits and reduced cost-sharing you get through the Marketplace will stop.

Where can I get more information?

To learn more about how Medicare works with the Marketplace, visit HealthCare.gov and Medicare.gov.

How much does Part A coverage cost?

You usually don't pay a monthly premium for Part A coverage if you or your spouse paid Medicare taxes while working. This is sometimes called premium-free Part A. If you aren't eligible for premium-free Part A, you may be able to buy Part A if:

- You're 65 or older, and you have (or are enrolling in) Part B and meet the citizenship and residency requirements.

- You're under 65, disabled, and your premium-free Part A coverage ended because you returned to work. (If you're under 65 and disabled, you can continue to get premium-free Part A for up to 8 1/2 years after you return to work.)

Note: In 2014, people who had to buy Part A paid up to $426 each month. Visit Medicare.gov, or call 1-800-MEDICARE (1-800-633-4227) to find out the amount for 2015. TTY users should call 1-877-486-2048.

Definitions of blue words are on pages 145–148.

In most cases, if you choose to **buy** Part A, you must also have Part B and pay monthly premiums for both. If you have limited income and resources, your state may help you pay for Part A and/or Part B. See pages 115–116. Call Social Security at 1-800-772-1213 for more information about the Part A premium. TTY users should call 1-800-325-0778.

What's the Part A late enrollment penalty?

If you aren't eligible for premium-free Part A, and you don't buy it when you're first eligible, your monthly premium may go up 10% when you decide to enroll. You'll have to pay the higher premium for twice the number of years you could have had Part A, but didn't sign up.

> **Example:** If you were eligible for Part A for 2 years but didn't sign up, you'll have to pay the higher premium for 4 years. Usually, you don't have to pay a penalty if you meet certain conditions that allow you to sign up for Part A during a Special Enrollment Period. See pages 25–26.

How much does Part B coverage cost?

You pay the Part B premium each month. Most people will pay the standard premium amount, which was $104.90 in 2014. Visit Medicare.gov, or call 1-800-MEDICARE (1-800-633-4227) to find out the amount for 2015. TTY users should call 1-877-486-2048.

Some people may pay a higher Part B premium

If your modified adjusted gross income as reported on your IRS tax return from 2 years ago (the most recent tax return information provided to Social Security by the IRS) is above a certain amount ($85,000 if you file individually or $170,000 if you're married and file jointly), you may pay more. This doesn't affect everyone, so most people won't have to pay a higher amount. Your modified adjusted gross income is your adjusted gross income plus your tax exempt interest income.

Each year, Social Security will tell you if you have to pay more than the standard premium. The amount you pay can change each year depending on your income. If you have to pay a higher amount for your Part B premium and you disagree (for example, if your income goes down), call Social Security at 1-800-772-1213. TTY users should call 1-800-325-0778. If you get benefits from RRB, you should still contact Social Security because the RRB doesn't make income determinations. For more information, visit socialsecurity.gov/pubs/EN-05-10536.pdf to view the fact sheet "Medicare Premiums: Rules for Higher-Income Beneficiaries."

What's the Part B late enrollment penalty?

If you don't sign up for Part B when you're first eligible, you may have to pay a late enrollment penalty for as long as you have Part B. Your monthly premium for Part B may go up 10% for each full 12-month period that you could have had Part B, but didn't sign up for it. Usually, you don't pay a late enrollment penalty if you meet certain conditions that allow you to sign up for Part B during a Special Enrollment Period. See pages 25–26.

> **Example:** Mr. Smith's Initial Enrollment Period ended September 30, 2011. He waited to sign up for Part B until March 2014 during the General Enrollment Period. His Part B premium penalty is 20%. (Even though Mr. Smith waited a total of 30 months to sign up, this included only 2 full 12-month periods.) He'll have to pay this penalty for as long as he has Part B.

If you have limited income and resources, see pages 115–116 for information about help paying your Medicare premiums.

How can I pay my Part B premium?

If you get Social Security, RRB, or Office of Personnel Management (OPM) benefits, your Part B premium will be automatically deducted from your benefit payment. If you don't get these benefit payments and choose to sign up for Part B, you'll get a bill. If you choose to buy Part A, you'll always get a bill for your premium. There are 3 ways to pay these bills:

1. Mail your premium payments to:

   Medicare Premium Collection Center
   P.O. Box 790355
   St. Louis, Missouri 63179-0355

   If you get a bill from the RRB, mail your premium payments to:

   RRB
   Medicare Premium Payments
   P.O. Box 979024
   St. Louis, Missouri 63197-9000

2. Pay by credit card. To do this, complete the bottom portion of the payment coupon on your Medicare bill and mail it to the address above.

3. Sign up for Medicare Easy Pay, a free service that automatically deducts your premium payments from your savings or checking account each month. Visit Medicare.gov to learn more and to find out how to sign up.

If you have questions about your premiums, call Social Security at 1-800-772-1213. TTY users should call 1-800-325-0778. If your bills are from the RRB, call 1-877-772-5772. TTY users should call 1-312-751-4701.

Definitions of blue words are on pages 145–148.

Section 3—

Find Out if Medicare Covers Your Test, Service, or Item

What services does Medicare cover?

Medicare covers certain medical services and supplies in hospitals, doctors' offices, and other health care settings. Services are either covered under Part A or Part B.

If you have both Part A and Part B, you can get all of the Medicare-covered services listed in this section, whether you have Original Medicare or a Medicare Advantage Plan.

Important! To get Medicare-covered Part A and/or Part B services, you must be a U.S. citizen or be lawfully present in the U.S.

What does Part A cover?

Part A (Hospital Insurance) helps cover:

- Inpatient care in hospitals
- Inpatient care in a skilled nursing facility (not custodial or long-term care)
- Hospice care
- Home health care
- Inpatient care in a religious nonmedical health care institution

You can find out if you have Part A by looking at your red, white, and blue Medicare card. If you have Original Medicare, you'll use this card to get your Medicare-covered services. If you join a Medicare Advantage Plan, in most cases, you must use the card from the plan to get your Medicare-covered services.

What do I pay for Part A-covered services?

Copayments, coinsurance, or deductibles may apply for each service listed on the following pages. Visit Medicare.gov, or call 1-800-MEDICARE (1-800-633-4227) to get specific cost information. TTY users should call 1-877-486-2048.

If you're in a Medicare Advantage Plan or have other insurance (like a Medicare Supplement Insurance (Medigap) policy, or employer or union coverage), your costs may be different. Contact the plans you're interested in to find out about the costs, or visit the Medicare Plan Finder at Medicare.gov/find-a-plan.

> Definitions of blue words are on pages 145–148.

Part A-covered services

Blood

If the hospital gets blood from a blood bank at no charge, you won't have to pay for it or replace it. If the hospital has to buy blood for you, you must either pay the hospital costs for the first 3 units of blood you get in a calendar year or have the blood donated by you or someone else.

Home health services

Medicare covers medically necessary part-time or intermittent skilled nursing care, and/or physical therapy, speech-language pathology services, and/or services for people with a continuing need for occupational therapy. A doctor, or certain health care professionals who work with a doctor, must see you face-to-face before a doctor can certify that you need home health services. A doctor must order your care, and a Medicare-certified home health agency must provide it. Home health services may also include medical social services, part-time or intermittent home health aide services, and medical supplies for use at home. You must be homebound, which means both of these are true:

1. You're normally unable to leave home and doing so requires a considerable and taxing effort.

2. Because of an illness or injury, leaving home isn't medically advisable or isn't possible without the aid of supportive devices, use of special transportation, or the assistance of another person.

You pay nothing for covered home health care services and 20% of the Medicare-approved amount for durable medical equipment. See pages 47–48.

Hospice care

To qualify for hospice care, a hospice doctor and your doctor (if you have one) must certify that you're terminally ill, meaning you have a life expectancy of 6 months or less. If you're already getting hospice care, a hospice doctor or nurse practitioner will need to see you about 6 months after your hospice care started to certify that you're still terminally ill. Coverage includes:

- All items and services needed for pain relief and symptom management
- Medical, nursing, and social services
- Drugs
- Certain durable medical equipment
- Aide and homemaker services
- Other covered services, as well as services Medicare usually doesn't cover, like spiritual and grief counseling

A Medicare-approved hospice usually gives hospice care in your home or other facility where you live, like a nursing home.

Hospice care doesn't pay for your stay in a facility (room and board) unless the hospice medical team determines that you need short-term inpatient stays for pain and symptom management that can't be addressed at home. These stays must be in a Medicare-approved facility, like a hospice facility, hospital, or skilled nursing facility that contracts with the hospice. Medicare also covers inpatient respite care, which is care you get in a Medicare-approved facility so that your usual caregiver can rest. You can stay up to 5 days each time you get respite care. Medicare will pay for covered services for health problems that aren't related to your terminal illness or related conditions. You can continue to get hospice care as long as the hospice medical director or hospice doctor recertifies that you're terminally ill.

- You pay nothing for hospice care.
- You pay a copayment of up to $5 per prescription for outpatient prescription drugs for pain and symptom management. In the rare case your drug isn't covered by the hospice benefit, your hospice provider should contact your Medicare drug plan to see if it's covered under Part D.
- You pay 5% of the Medicare-approved amount for inpatient respite care.

Hospital care (inpatient care)

Medicare covers semi-private rooms, meals, general nursing, and drugs as part of your inpatient treatment, and other hospital services and supplies. This includes care you get in acute care hospitals, critical access hospitals, inpatient rehabilitation facilities, long-term care hospitals, inpatient care as part of a qualifying clinical research study, and mental health care. This doesn't include private-duty nursing, a television or phone in your room (if there's a separate charge for these items), or personal care items, like razors or slipper socks. It also doesn't include a private room, unless medically necessary. If you have Part B, it covers the doctor's services you get while you're in a hospital.

> Definitions of blue words are on pages 145–148.

- You pay a deductible and no coinsurance for days 1–60 of each benefit period.
- You pay coinsurance for days 61–90 of each benefit period.
- You pay coinsurance per "lifetime reserve day" after day 90 of each benefit period (up to 60 days over your lifetime).
- You pay all costs for each day after you use all the lifetime reserve days.
- Inpatient psychiatric care in a freestanding psychiatric hospital is limited to 190 days in a lifetime.

Are you an inpatient?

Important!

Staying overnight in a hospital doesn't always mean you're an inpatient. You only become an inpatient when a hospital formally admits you as an inpatient, after a doctor orders it. You're still an outpatient if you haven't been formally admitted as an inpatient, even if you're getting emergency department services, observation services, outpatient surgery, lab tests, or X-rays. **You or a family member should always ask if you're an inpatient or an outpatient each day during your stay, since it affects what you pay and can affect whether you'll qualify for Part A coverage in a skilled nursing facility.**

For more information, visit Medicare.gov/publications to view the fact sheet "Are You a Hospital Inpatient or Outpatient? If You Have Medicare—Ask!"

Religious non-medical health care institution (inpatient care)

In these facilities, religious beliefs prohibit conventional and unconventional medical care. If you qualify for hospital or skilled nursing facility care, Medicare will only cover the inpatient, non-religious, non-medical items and services. An example is room and board, or any items and services that don't require a doctor's order or prescription, like unmedicated wound dressings or use of a simple walker.

Skilled nursing facility care

Medicare covers semi-private rooms, meals, skilled nursing and rehabilitative services, and other medically necessary services

and supplies after a 3-day minimum, medically necessary, inpatient hospital stay for a related illness or injury. An inpatient hospital stay begins the day the hospital formally admits you as an inpatient based on a doctor's order and doesn't include the day you're discharged. To qualify for care in a skilled nursing facility, your doctor must certify that you need daily skilled care like intravenous injections or physical therapy. Medicare doesn't cover long-term care or custodial care.

- You pay nothing for the first 20 days of each benefit period.
- You pay a coinsurance per day for days 21–100 of each benefit period.
- You pay all costs for each day after day 100 in a benefit period.

Note: Visit Medicare.gov, or call 1-800-MEDICARE (1-800-633-4227) to find out what you pay for inpatient hospital stays and skilled nursing facility care in 2015. TTY users should call 1-877-486-2048.

What does Part B cover?

Medicare Part B (Medical Insurance) helps cover medically necessary doctors' services, outpatient care, home health services, durable medical equipment, and other medical services. Part B also covers many preventive services. You can find out if you have Part B by looking at your red, white, and blue Medicare card. See pages 41–60 for a list of common Part B-covered services and general descriptions. Medicare may cover some services and tests more often than the timeframes listed if needed to diagnose or treat a condition. To find out if Medicare covers a service not on this list, visit Medicare.gov/coverage, or call 1-800-MEDICARE (1-800-633-4227). TTY users should call 1-877-486-2048. For more details about Medicare covered services, visit Medicare.gov/publications to view the booklet "Your Medicare Benefits." Call 1-800-MEDICARE to find out if a copy can be mailed to you.

What do I pay for Part B-covered services?

The alphabetical list on the following pages gives general information about what you pay if you have Original Medicare and see doctors or other health care providers who accept assignment. See pages 70–71. You'll pay more if you see doctors or providers who don't accept assignment. **If you're in a Medicare Advantage Plan (like an HMO or PPO) or have other insurance, your costs may be different. Contact your plan or benefits administrator directly to find out about the costs.**

Definitions of blue words are on pages 145–148.

Under Original Medicare, if the Part B deductible applies, you must pay all costs (up to the Medicare-approved amount) until you meet the yearly Part B deductible before Medicare begins to pay its share. Then, after your deductible is met, you typically pay 20% of the Medicare-approved amount of the service, if the doctor or other health care provider accepts assignment. There's no yearly limit for what you pay out-of-pocket. Visit Medicare.gov or call 1-800-MEDICARE to get specific cost information.

You pay nothing for most covered preventive services if you get the services from a doctor or other qualified health care provider who accepts assignment. However, for some preventive services, you may have to pay a deductible, coinsurance, or both. These costs may also apply if you get a preventive service in the same visit as a non-preventive service.

Part B-covered services

You'll see this apple next to the preventive services on pages 41–60. Use the preventive services checklist on page 61 to ask your doctor or other health care provider which preventive services you should get.

Abdominal aortic aneurysm screening

Medicare covers a one-time screening abdominal aortic aneurysm ultrasound for people at risk. You must get a referral from your doctor or other practitioner. You pay nothing for the screening if the doctor or other qualified health care provider accepts assignment.

Note: If you have a family history of abdominal aortic aneurysms, or you're a man 65–75 and you've smoked at least 100 cigarettes in your lifetime, you're considered at risk.

Alcohol misuse screening and counseling

Medicare covers one alcohol misuse screening per year for adults with Medicare (including pregnant women) who use alcohol, but don't meet the medical criteria for alcohol dependency. If your primary care doctor or other primary care practitioner determines you're misusing alcohol, you can get up to 4 brief face-to-face counseling sessions per year (if you're competent and alert during counseling). A qualified primary care doctor or other primary care practitioner must provide the counseling in a primary care setting (like a doctor's office). You pay nothing if the qualified primary care doctor or other primary care practitioner accepts assignment.

Ambulance services

Medicare covers ground ambulance transportation when you need to be transported to a hospital, critical access hospital, or skilled nursing facility for medically necessary services, and transportation in any other vehicle could endanger your health. Medicare may pay for emergency ambulance transportation in an airplane or helicopter to a hospital if you need immediate and rapid ambulance transportation that ground transportation can't provide. In some cases, Medicare may pay for limited, medically necessary, non-emergency ambulance transportation if you have a written order from your doctor stating that ambulance transportation is necessary due to your medical condition. Medicare will only cover ambulance services to the nearest appropriate medical facility that's able to give you the care you need. You pay 20% of the Medicare-approved amount, and the Part B deductible applies.

> Definitions of blue words are on pages 145–148.

Ambulatory surgical centers

Medicare covers the facility service fees related to approved surgical procedures in an ambulatory surgical center (facility where surgical procedures are performed), and the patient is expected to be released within 24 hours. Except for certain preventive services (for which you pay nothing if the doctor or other health care provider accepts assignment), you pay 20% of the Medicare-approved amount to both the ambulatory surgical center and the doctor who treats you, and the Part B deductible applies. You pay all of the facility service fees for procedures Medicare doesn't cover in ambulatory surgical centers.

Blood

If the provider gets blood from a blood bank at no charge, you won't have to pay for it or replace it. However, you'll pay a copayment for the blood processing and handling services for each unit of blood you get, and the Part B deductible applies. If the provider has to buy blood for you, you must either pay the provider costs for the first 3 units of blood you get in a calendar year or have the blood donated by you or someone else.

Bone mass measurement (bone density)

This test helps to see if you're at risk for broken bones. It's covered once every 24 months (more often if medically necessary) for people who have certain medical conditions or meet certain criteria. You pay nothing for this test if the doctor or other qualified health care provider accepts assignment.

Breast cancer screening (mammograms)

Medicare covers screening mammograms to check for breast cancer once every 12 months for all women with Medicare who are 40 and older. Medicare covers one baseline mammogram for women between 35–39. You pay nothing for the test if the doctor or other qualified health care provider accepts assignment.

Cardiac rehabilitation

Medicare covers comprehensive programs that include exercise, education, and counseling for patients who meet these conditions:

- A heart attack in the last 12 months
- Coronary artery bypass surgery
- Current stable angina pectoris (chest pain)
- A heart valve repair or replacement
- A coronary angioplasty (a medical procedure used to open a blocked artery) or coronary stenting (a procedure used to keep an artery open)
- A heart or heart-lung transplant

Medicare also covers intensive cardiac rehabilitation programs that are typically more rigorous or more intense than regular cardiac rehabilitation programs. Services are covered in a doctor's office or hospital outpatient setting. You pay 20% of the Medicare-approved amount if you get the services in a doctor's office. In a hospital outpatient setting, you also pay the hospital a copayment. The Part B deductible applies.

Cardiovascular disease (behavioral therapy)

Medicare will cover one visit per year with a primary care doctor in a primary care setting (like a doctor's office) to help lower your risk for cardiovascular disease. During this visit, the doctor may discuss aspirin use (if appropriate), check your blood pressure, and give you tips to make sure you're eating well. You pay nothing if the doctor or other qualified health care provider accepts assignment.

Cardiovascular disease screenings

These screenings include blood tests that help detect conditions that may lead to a heart attack or stroke. Medicare covers these screening tests once every 5 years to test your cholesterol, lipid, lipoprotein, and triglyceride levels. You pay nothing for the tests if the doctor or other qualified health care provider accepts assignment.

Cervical and vaginal cancer screening

Medicare covers Pap tests and pelvic exams to check for cervical and vaginal cancers. As part of the exam, Medicare also covers a clinical breast exam to check for breast cancer. Medicare covers these screening tests once every 24 months. Medicare covers these screening tests once every 12 months if you're at high risk for cervical or vaginal cancer or if you're of child-bearing age and had an abnormal Pap test in the past 36 months. You pay nothing if the doctor or other qualified health care provider accepts assignment.

Chemotherapy

Medicare covers chemotherapy in a doctor's office, freestanding clinic, or hospital outpatient setting for people with cancer. You pay a copayment for chemotherapy in a hospital outpatient setting.

For chemotherapy given in a doctor's office or freestanding clinic, you pay 20% of the Medicare-approved amount, and the Part B deductible applies.

For chemotherapy in a hospital inpatient setting covered under Part A, see Hospital care (inpatient care) on page 38.

Chiropractic services (limited coverage)

Medicare covers manipulation of the spine if medically necessary to correct a subluxation (when one or more of the bones of your spine move out of position) when provided by a chiropractor or other qualified provider. You pay 20% of the Medicare-approved amount, and the Part B deductible applies.

Note: You pay all costs for any other services or tests ordered by a chiropractor (including X-rays and massage therapy).

Definitions of blue words are on pages 145–148.

Clinical research studies

Clinical research studies test how well different types of medical care work and if they're safe. Medicare covers some costs, like office visits and tests, in qualifying clinical research studies. You may pay 20% of the Medicare-approved amount, and the Part B deductible may apply.

Note: If you're in a Medicare Advantage Plan (like an HMO or PPO), some costs may be covered by Medicare and some may be covered by your plan.

Colorectal cancer screenings

Medicare covers these screenings to help find precancerous growths or find cancer early, when treatment is most effective. One or more of these tests may be covered:

- **Screening fecal occult blood test**—This test is covered once every 12 months if you're 50 or older. You pay nothing for the test if the doctor or other qualified health care provider accepts assignment.
- **Screening flexible sigmoidoscopy**—This test is generally covered once every 48 months if you're 50 or older, or 120 months after a previous screening colonoscopy for those not at high risk. You pay nothing for the test if the doctor or other qualified health care provider accepts assignment.
- **Screening colonoscopy**—This test is generally covered once every 120 months (high risk every 24 months) or 48 months after a previous flexible sigmoidoscopy. There's no minimum age. You pay nothing for the test if the doctor or other qualified health care provider accepts assignment.
  Note: If a polyp or other tissue is found and removed during the colonoscopy, you may have to pay 20% of the Medicare-approved amount for the doctor's services and a copayment in a hospital outpatient setting. The Part B deductible doesn't apply.
- **Screening barium enema**—This test is generally covered once every 48 months if you're 50 or older (high risk every 24 months) when used instead of a sigmoidoscopy or colonoscopy. You pay 20% of the Medicare-approved amount for the doctor services. In a hospital outpatient setting, you also pay the hospital a copayment.

Defibrillator (implantable automatic)

Medicare covers these devices for some people diagnosed with heart failure. If the surgery takes place in an outpatient setting, you pay 20% of the Medicare-approved amount for the doctor's services. If you get the device as a hospital outpatient, you also pay the hospital a copayment. In most cases, the copayment amount can't be more than the Part A hospital stay deductible. The Part B deductible applies. Surgeries to implant defibrillators in a hospital inpatient setting are covered under Part A. See Hospital care (inpatient care) on page 38.

Depression screening

Medicare covers one depression screening per year. The screening must be done in a primary care setting (like a doctor's office) that can provide follow-up treatment and referrals. You pay nothing for this test if the doctor or other qualified health care provider accepts assignment.

Diabetes screenings

Medicare covers these screenings if your doctor determines you're at risk for diabetes. You may be eligible for up to 2 diabetes screenings each year. You pay nothing for the test if your doctor or other qualified health care provider accepts assignment.

Diabetes self-management training

Medicare covers diabetes outpatient self-management training to teach you to cope with and manage your diabetes. The program may include tips for eating healthy, being active, monitoring blood sugar, taking medication, and reducing risks. You must have diabetes and a written order from your doctor or other health care provider. You pay 20% of the Medicare-approved amount, and the Part B deductible applies.

Definitions of blue words are on pages 145–148.

Diabetes supplies

Medicare covers blood sugar testing monitors, blood sugar test strips, lancet devices and lancets, blood sugar control solutions, and therapeutic shoes (in some cases). Medicare only covers insulin if it's medically necessary and you use an external insulin pump to administer the insulin. You pay 20% of the Medicare-approved amount, and the Part B deductible applies.

Note: Medicare prescription drug coverage (Part D) may cover insulin, certain medical supplies used to inject insulin (like syringes), and some oral diabetic drugs. Check with your plan for more information.

Important!

You may need to use specific suppliers for some types of diabetic testing supplies. Visit Medicare.gov/supplierdirectory to find a list of suppliers for your area.

Doctor and other health care provider services

Medicare covers medically necessary doctor services (including outpatient services and some doctor services you get when you're a hospital inpatient) and covered preventive services. Medicare also covers services provided by other health care providers, like physician assistants, nurse practitioners, social workers, physical therapists, and psychologists. Except for certain preventive services (for which you may pay nothing), you pay 20% of the Medicare-approved amount, and the Part B deductible applies.

Durable medical equipment (like walkers)

Medicare covers items like oxygen equipment and supplies, wheelchairs, walkers, and hospital beds ordered by a doctor or other health care provider enrolled in Medicare for use in the home. Some items must be rented. You pay 20% of the Medicare-approved amount, and the Part B deductible applies. **In all areas of the country, you must get your covered equipment or supplies and replacement or repair services from a Medicare-approved supplier for Medicare to pay.**

For more information, visit Medicare.gov/publications to view the booklet "Medicare Coverage of Durable Medical Equipment and Other Devices." You can also call 1-800-MEDICARE (1-800-633-4227) to find out if a copy can be mailed to you. TTY users should call 1-877-486-2048.

Durable Medical Equipment, Prosthetics, Orthotics, and Supplies (DMEPOS) Competitive Bidding Program: If you have Original Medicare and live in a Competitive Bidding Area (CBA) and use equipment or supplies included under the program (or get the items while visiting a CBA), you generally must use Medicare contract suppliers if you want Medicare to help pay for the item. Visit Medicare.gov/supplier to determine if you live in a CBA and to find Medicare-approved suppliers in your area. If your ZIP code is in a CBA, the items included in the program are marked with an orange star. You can also call 1-800-MEDICARE.

The competitive bidding program applies to Original Medicare only. If you're enrolled in a Medicare Advantage Plan (like an HMO or PPO), your plan will notify you if your supplier is changing. If you're not sure, contact your plan.

> Definitions of blue words are on pages 145–148.

EKG or ECG (electrocardiogram) screening

Medicare covers a one-time screening EKG/ECG if referred by your doctor or other health care provider as part of your one-time "Welcome to Medicare" preventive visit. See pages 59–60. You pay 20% of the Medicare-approved amount, and the Part B deductible applies. An EKG/ECG is also covered as a diagnostic test. See page 57. If you have the test at a hospital or a hospital-owned clinic, you also pay the hospital a copayment.

Emergency department services

These services are covered when you have an injury, a sudden illness, or an illness that quickly gets much worse. You pay a specified copayment for the hospital emergency department visit, and you pay 20% of the Medicare-approved amount for the doctor's or other health care provider's services. The Part B deductible applies. However, your costs may be different if you're admitted to the hospital.

Eyeglasses (limited)

Medicare covers one pair of eyeglasses with standard frames (or one set of contact lenses) after cataract surgery that implants an intraocular lens. You pay 20% of the Medicare-approved amount, and the Part B deductible applies. **Note:** Medicare will only pay for contact lenses or eyeglasses from a supplier enrolled in Medicare.

Federally qualified health center services

Federally qualified health centers (FQHCs) furnish many outpatient primary care and preventive health services. There's no deductible, and generally, you're responsible for paying 20% of your charges or 20% of the Medicare-approved amount, except for most preventive services for which there's no copayment required. All FQHCs offer a sliding fee schedule to persons with incomes below 200% of the Federal poverty level. To find a FQHC near you, visit findahealthcenter.hrsa.gov.

Flu shots

Medicare generally covers one flu shot per flu season. You pay nothing for the flu shot if the doctor or other qualified health care provider accepts assignment for giving the shot.

Foot exams and treatment

Medicare covers foot exams and treatment if you have diabetes-related nerve damage and/or meet certain conditions. You pay 20% of the Medicare-approved amount, and the Part B deductible applies. In a hospital outpatient setting, you also pay the hospital a copayment.

Glaucoma tests

These tests are covered once every 12 months for people at high risk for the eye disease glaucoma. You're at high risk if you have diabetes, a family history of glaucoma, are African-American and 50 or older, or are Hispanic and 65 or older. An eye doctor who's legally allowed by the state must do the tests. You pay 20% of the Medicare-approved amount, and the Part B deductible applies. In a hospital outpatient setting, you also pay the hospital a copayment.

Hearing and balance exams

Medicare covers these exams if your doctor or other health care provider orders them to see if you need medical treatment. You pay 20% of the Medicare-approved amount, and the Part B deductible applies. In a hospital outpatient setting, you also pay the hospital a copayment.

Note: Original Medicare doesn't cover hearing aids or exams for fitting hearing aids.

Hepatitis B shots

Medicare covers these shots for people at medium or high risk for Hepatitis B. Some risk factors include hemophilia, End-Stage Renal Disease (ESRD), diabetes, if you live with someone who has Hepatitis B, or if you're a health care worker and have frequent contact with blood or body fluids. Check with your doctor to see if you're at medium or high risk for Hepatitis B. You pay nothing for getting the shot if the doctor or other qualified health care provider accepts assignment.

HIV screening

Medicare covers HIV (Human Immunodeficiency Virus) screenings for people with Medicare at increased risk for the virus, people who ask for the test, or pregnant women. Medicare covers this test once every 12 months or up to 3 times during a pregnancy. You pay nothing for the HIV screening if the doctor or other qualified health care provider accepts assignment.

Home health services

Medicare covers medically necessary part-time or intermittent skilled nursing care, and/or physical therapy, speech-language pathology services, and/or services for people with a continuing need for occupational therapy. A doctor, or certain health care professionals who work with a doctor, must see you face-to-face before a doctor can certify that you need home health services. A doctor must order your care, and a Medicare-certified home health agency must provide it.

Home health services may also include medical social services, part-time or intermittent home health aide services, durable medical equipment, and medical supplies for use at home. You must be homebound, which means both of these are true:

1. You have trouble leaving your home without help (like using a cane, wheelchair, walker, or crutches; special transportation; or help from another person) because of an illness or injury.

2. Leaving your home isn't recommended because of your condition, and you're normally unable to leave your home because it's a major effort.

You pay nothing for covered home health services. For Medicare-covered durable medical equipment information, see pages 47–48.

Kidney dialysis services and supplies

Generally, Medicare covers 3 dialysis treatments per week if you have End-Stage Renal Disease (ESRD). This includes all ESRD-related drugs and biologicals, laboratory tests, home dialysis training, support services, equipment, and supplies. The dialysis facility is responsible for coordinating your dialysis services (at home or in a facility). You pay 20% of the Medicare-approved amount, and the Part B deductible applies.

Kidney disease education services

Medicare covers up to 6 sessions of kidney disease education services if you have Stage IV chronic kidney disease, and your doctor or other health care provider refers you for the service. You pay 20% of the Medicare-approved amount, and the Part B deductible applies.

Laboratory services

Medicare covers laboratory services including certain blood tests, urinalysis, and some screening tests. You generally pay nothing for these services.

Definitions of blue words are on pages 145–148.

Medical nutrition therapy services

Medicare may cover medical nutrition therapy and certain related services if you have diabetes or kidney disease, or you have had a kidney transplant in the last 36 months, and your doctor or other health care provider refers you for the service. You pay nothing for these services if the doctor or other qualified health care provider accepts assignment.

Mental health care (outpatient)

Medicare covers mental health care services to help with conditions like depression or anxiety. Coverage includes services generally provided in an outpatient setting (like a doctor's or other health care provider's office or hospital outpatient department), including visits with a psychiatrist or other doctor, clinical psychologist, nurse practitioner, physician assistant, clinical nurse specialist, or clinical social worker. Laboratory tests are also covered. Certain limits and conditions apply.

Generally, you pay 20% of the Medicare-approved amount and the Part B deductible applies for:

- Visits to a doctor or other health care provider to diagnose your condition or monitor or change your prescriptions
- Outpatient treatment of your condition (like counseling or psychotherapy)

Note: Inpatient mental health care is covered under Part A. See Hospital care (inpatient care) on page 38.

Obesity screening and counseling

If you have a body mass index (BMI) of 30 or more, Medicare may cover up to 22 face-to-face intensive counseling sessions over a 12-month period to help you lose weight. This counseling is covered when provided in a primary care setting (like a doctor's office). Talk to your primary care doctor or primary care practitioner to find out more. You pay nothing for this service if the primary care doctor or other qualified primary care practitioner accepts assignment.

Occupational therapy

Medicare covers evaluation and treatment to help you perform activities of daily living (like dressing or bathing) when your doctor or other health care provider certifies you need it. There may be a limit on the amount Medicare will pay for these services in a single year, and there may be certain exceptions to these limits. You pay 20% of the Medicare-approved amount, and the Part B deductible applies.

Outpatient hospital services

Medicare covers many diagnostic and treatment services in participating hospital outpatient departments. Generally, you pay 20% of the Medicare-approved amount for the doctor's or other health care provider's services. You may pay more for services you get in a hospital outpatient setting than you'll pay for the same care in a doctor's office. In addition to the amount you pay the doctor, you'll usually pay the hospital a copayment for each service you get in a hospital outpatient setting, except for certain preventive services that don't have a copayment. In most cases the copayment can't be more than the Part A hospital stay deductible for each service. The Part B deductible applies, except for certain preventive services. If you get hospital outpatient services in a critical access hospital, your copayment may be higher and may exceed the Part A hospital stay deductible.

Outpatient medical and surgical services and supplies

Medicare covers approved procedures like X-rays, casts, stitches, or outpatient surgeries. You pay 20% of the Medicare-approved amount for the doctor's or other health care provider's services. You generally pay the hospital a copayment for each service you get in a hospital outpatient setting. In most cases, for each service provided, the copayment can't be more than the Part A hospital stay deductible. The Part B deductible applies, and you pay all charges for items or services that Medicare doesn't cover.

Definitions of blue words are on pages 145–148.

Physical therapy

Medicare covers evaluation and treatment for injuries and diseases that change your ability to function when your doctor or other health care provider certifies your need for it. There may be a limit on the amount Medicare will pay for these services in a single year, and there may be certain exceptions to these limits. You pay 20% of the Medicare-approved amount, and the Part B deductible applies.

Pneumococcal shot

Medicare covers pneumococcal shots to help prevent pneumococcal infections (like certain types of pneumonia). Most people only need this shot once in their lifetime. Talk with your doctor or other health care provider to see if you should get this shot. You pay nothing for getting the shot if the doctor or other qualified health care provider accepts assignment for giving the shot.

Prescription drugs (limited)

Medicare covers a limited number of drugs like injections you get in a doctor's office, certain oral anti-cancer drugs, drugs used with some types of durable medical equipment (like a nebulizer or external infusion pump), immunosuppressant drugs (see page 58), and under very limited circumstances, certain drugs you get in a hospital outpatient setting. You pay 20% of the Medicare-approved amount for these covered drugs, and the Part B deductible applies.

Definitions of blue words are on pages 145–148.

If the covered drugs you get in a hospital outpatient setting are part of your outpatient services, you pay a copayment for the services. However, other types of drugs in a hospital outpatient setting (sometimes called "self-administered drugs" or drugs you would normally take on your own) aren't covered by Part B. What you pay depends on whether you have Part D or other prescription drug coverage, whether your drug plan covers the drug, and whether the hospital's pharmacy is in your drug plan's network. Contact your prescription drug plan to find out what you pay for drugs you get in a hospital outpatient setting that aren't covered under Part B.

Other than the examples above, you pay 100% for most prescription drugs, unless you have Part D or other drug coverage. See pages 97–110 for more information about Part D.

Prostate cancer screenings

Medicare covers a Prostate Specific Antigen (PSA) test and a digital rectal exam once every 12 months for men over 50 (beginning the day after your 50th birthday). You pay nothing for the PSA test. You pay 20% of the Medicare-approved amount, and the Part B deductible applies for the digital rectal exam. In a hospital outpatient setting, you also pay the hospital a copayment.

Prosthetic/orthotic items

Medicare covers arm, leg, back, and neck braces; artificial eyes; artificial limbs (and their replacement parts); some types of breast prostheses (after mastectomy); and prosthetic devices needed to replace an internal body part or function (including ostomy supplies, and parenteral and enteral nutrition therapy) when ordered by a doctor or other health care provider enrolled in Medicare.

For Medicare to cover your prosthetic or orthotic, you must go to a supplier that's enrolled in Medicare. You pay 20% of the Medicare-approved amount, and the Part B deductible applies.

Important!

DMEPOS Competitive Bidding Program: To get enteral nutrition therapy in most areas of the country, you generally must use specific suppliers called "contract suppliers," or Medicare won't pay and you'll likely pay full price. See page 48 for more information.

Pulmonary rehabilitation

Medicare covers a comprehensive pulmonary rehabilitation program if you have moderate to very severe chronic obstructive pulmonary disease (COPD) and have a referral from the doctor treating this chronic respiratory disease. You pay 20% of the Medicare-approved amount if you get the service in a doctor's office. You also pay the hospital a copayment per session if you get the service in a hospital outpatient setting. The Part B deductible applies.

Rural health clinic services

Rural health clinics (RHCs) furnish many outpatient primary care and preventive health services. Generally, you're responsible for paying 20% of the charges, except for most preventive services for which there's no copayment required. RHCs are located in non-urban areas that are medically underserved or shortage areas.

Second surgical opinions

Medicare covers second surgical opinions in some cases for surgery that isn't an emergency. In some cases, Medicare covers third surgical opinions. You pay 20% of the Medicare-approved amount, and the Part B deductible applies.

Sexually transmitted infections screening and counseling

Medicare covers sexually transmitted infection (STI) screenings for chlamydia, gonorrhea, syphilis, and Hepatitis B. These screenings are covered for people with Medicare who are pregnant and for certain people who are at increased risk for an STI when the tests are ordered by a primary care doctor or other primary care practitioner. Medicare covers these tests once every 12 months or at certain times during pregnancy.

Medicare also covers up to 2 individual, 20–30 minute, face-to-face, high-intensity behavioral counseling sessions each year for sexually active adults at increased risk for STIs. Medicare will only cover these counseling sessions if they're provided by a primary care doctor or other primary care practitioner and take place in a primary care setting (like a doctor's office). Counseling conducted in an inpatient setting, like a skilled nursing facility, won't be covered as a preventive service.

You pay nothing for these services if the primary care doctor or other qualified primary care practitioner accepts assignment.

Shots

Part B covers:

Flu shots. See page 49.
Hepatitis B shots. See page 50.
Pneumococcal shots. See page 54.

Note about the shingles shot:

The shingles shot isn't covered by Part A or Part B. Generally, Medicare prescription drug plans (Part D) cover all commercially available vaccines (like the shingles shot) needed to prevent illness. Contact your Medicare drug plan for more information about coverage.

Speech-language pathology services

Medicare covers evaluation and treatment given to regain and strengthen speech and language skills, including cognitive and swallowing skills, when your doctor or other health care provider certifies you need it. There may be a limit on the amount Medicare will pay for these services in a single year, and there may be certain exceptions to these limits. You pay 20% of the Medicare-approved amount, and the Part B deductible applies.

Surgical dressing services

Medicare covers these services for treatment of a surgical or surgically treated wound. You pay 20% of the Medicare-approved amount for the doctor's or other health care provider's services. You pay a fixed copayment for these services when you get them in a hospital outpatient setting. You pay nothing for the supplies, and the Part B deductible applies.

Telehealth

Medicare covers limited medical or other health services like office visits and consultations provided using an interactive, two-way telecommunications system (like real-time audio and video) by an eligible provider who isn't at your location. These services are available in some rural areas, under certain conditions, and only if you're located at: a doctor's office, hospital, rural health clinic, federally qualified health center, hospital-based dialysis facility, skilled nursing facility, or community mental health center. For most of these services, you pay 20% of the Medicare-approved amount, and the Part B deductible applies.

Tests (other than lab tests)

Medicare covers X-rays, MRIs, CT scans, ECG/EKGs, and some other diagnostic tests. You pay 20% of the Medicare-approved amount, and the Part B deductible applies. If you get the test at a hospital as an outpatient, you also pay the hospital a copayment that may be more than 20% of the Medicare-approved amount, but in most cases, this amount can't be more than the Part A hospital stay deductible. See Laboratory services on page 51 for other Part B-covered tests.

Definitions of blue words are on pages 145–148.

Tobacco-use cessation counseling

If you use tobacco and you're diagnosed with an illness caused or complicated by tobacco use, or you take a medicine that's affected by tobacco, Medicare covers up to 8 face-to-face visits in a 12-month period. You pay 20% of the Medicare-approved amount, and the Part B deductible applies. In a hospital outpatient setting, you also pay the hospital a copayment.

If you haven't been diagnosed with an illness caused or complicated by tobacco use, Medicare coverage of tobacco use cessation counseling is considered a covered preventive service. Medicare covers up to 8 face-to-face visits in a 12-month period. You pay nothing for the counseling sessions if the doctor or other qualified health care provider accepts assignment.

Transplants and immunosuppressive drugs

Medicare covers doctor services for heart, lung, kidney, pancreas, intestine, and liver transplants under certain conditions and only in Medicare-certified facilities. Medicare covers bone marrow and cornea transplants under certain conditions.

Medicare covers immunosuppressive drugs if the transplant was covered by Medicare or an employer or union group health plan was required to pay before Medicare paid for the transplant. You must have Part A at the time of the covered transplant, and you must have Part B at the time you get immunosuppressive drugs. You pay 20% of the Medicare-approved amount for the drugs, and the Part B deductible applies.

If you're thinking about joining a Medicare Advantage Plan (like an HMO or PPO) and are on a transplant waiting list or believe you need a transplant, check with the plan before you join to make sure your doctors, other health care providers, and hospitals are in the plan's network. Also, check the plan's coverage rules for prior authorization.

Note: Medicare drug plans (Part D) may cover immunosuppressive drugs if they aren't covered by Original Medicare.

Definitions of blue words are on pages 145–148.

Travel (health care needed when traveling outside the U.S.)

Medicare generally doesn't cover health care while you're traveling outside the U.S. (The "U.S." includes the 50 states, the District of Columbia, Puerto Rico, the U.S. Virgin Islands, Guam, the Northern Mariana Islands, and American Samoa.) There are some exceptions, including cases where Medicare may pay for services that you get while on board a ship within the territorial waters adjoining the land areas of the U.S. Medicare may pay for inpatient hospital, doctor, or ambulance services you get in a foreign country in these rare cases:

1. You're in the U.S. when an emergency occurs, and the foreign hospital is closer than the nearest U.S. hospital that can treat your medical condition.

2. You're traveling through Canada without unreasonable delay by the most direct route between Alaska and another U.S. state when a medical emergency occurs, and the Canadian hospital is closer than the nearest U.S. hospital that can treat the emergency.

3. You live in the U.S. and the foreign hospital is closer to your home than the nearest U.S. hospital that can treat your medical condition, regardless of whether an emergency exists.

Medicare may cover medically necessary ambulance transportation to a foreign hospital only with admission for medically necessary covered inpatient hospital services. You pay 20% of the Medicare-approved amount, and the Part B deductible applies.

Urgently needed care

Medicare covers urgently needed care to treat a sudden illness or injury that isn't a medical emergency. You pay 20% of the Medicare-approved amount for the doctor's or other health care provider's services, and the Part B deductible applies. In a hospital outpatient setting, you also pay the hospital a copayment.

"Welcome to Medicare" preventive visit

During the first 12 months that you have Part B, you can get a "Welcome to Medicare" preventive visit. This visit includes a review of your medical and social history related to your health, and education and counseling about preventive services, including certain screenings, shots, and referrals for other care, if needed. When you make your appointment, let your doctor's office know that you would like to schedule your "Welcome to Medicare" preventive visit.

You pay nothing for the "Welcome to Medicare" preventive visit if the doctor or other qualified health care provider accepts assignment.

If your doctor or other health care provider performs additional tests or services during the same visit that aren't covered under this preventive benefit, you may have to pay coinsurance, and the Part B deductible may apply.

Yearly "Wellness" visit

If you've had Part B for longer than 12 months, you can get a yearly "Wellness" visit to develop or update a personalized plan to prevent disease or disability based on your current health and risk factors. This visit is covered once every 12 months.

Your provider will ask you to fill out a questionnaire, called a "Health Risk Assessment," as part of this visit. Answering these questions can help you and your provider develop a personalized prevention plan to help you stay healthy and get the most out of your visit. The questions are based on years of medical research and advice from the Centers for Disease Control and Prevention (CDC).

> Definitions of blue words are on pages 145–148.

When you make your appointment, let your doctor's office know that you would like to schedule your yearly "Wellness" visit.

Note: Your first yearly "Wellness" visit can't take place within 12 months of your enrollment in Part B or your "Welcome to Medicare" preventive visit. However, you don't need to have had a "Welcome to Medicare" preventive visit to qualify for a yearly "Wellness" visit.

You pay nothing for the yearly "Wellness" visit if the doctor or other qualified health care provider accepts assignment.

If your doctor or other health care provider performs additional tests or services during the same visit that aren't covered under this preventive benefit, you may have to pay coinsurance, and the Part B deductible may apply.

Want to keep track of your preventive services?

Medicare covers many preventive services to help you stay healthy. Talk with your health care provider about which of these services are right for you. You can also use Medicare's Blue Button to download your Original Medicare claim information. This will help you track the services you had and understand the services you might need. See page 135 for more information about the Blue Button. You can also visit bluebuttonconnector.healthit.gov to learn more about applications and services that are available to help you analyze your health information.

Page	Medicare-covered preventive service	I need (yes/no)
59	"Welcome to Medicare" preventive visit (one-time)	
60	Yearly "Wellness" visit	
41	Abdominal aortic aneurysm screening	
41	Alcohol misuse screening and counseling	
43	Bone mass measurement (bone density)	
43	Breast cancer screening (mammogram)	
43	Cardiovascular disease (behavioral therapy)	
44	Cardiovascular disease screenings	
44	Cervical and vaginal cancer screening	
45	Colorectal cancer screenings	
	Screening fecal occult blood test	
	Screening flexible sigmoidoscopy	
	Screening colonoscopy	
	Screening barium enema	

Page	Medicare-covered preventive service	I need (yes/no)
46	Depression screening	
46	Diabetes screenings	
46	Diabetes self-management training	
49	Flu shots	
49	Glaucoma tests	
50	Hepatitis B shots	
50	HIV screening	
52	Medical nutrition therapy services	
52	Obesity screening and counseling	
54	Pneumococcal shot	
55	Prostate cancer screenings	
56	Sexually transmitted infections screening and counseling	
58	Tobacco use cessation counseling (counseling for people with no sign of tobacco-related disease)	

What's NOT covered by Part A and Part B?

Medicare doesn't cover everything. If you need certain services that aren't covered under Medicare Part A or Part B, you'll have to pay for them yourself unless:

- You have other coverage (including Medicaid) to cover the costs.
- You're in a Medicare health plan that covers these services.

Even if Medicare covers a service or item, you generally have to pay deductibles, coinsurance, and copayments.

Some of the items and services that Medicare doesn't cover include:

- ✘ Most dental care.
- ✘ Eye examinations related to prescribing glasses.
- ✘ Dentures.
- ✘ Cosmetic surgery.
- ✘ Acupuncture.
- ✘ Hearing aids and exams for fitting them.
- ✘ Long-term care. See next page for more information about paying for long-term care.

Definitions of blue words are on pages 145–148.

If you have Original Medicare, visit Medicare.gov/coverage, or call 1-800-MEDICARE (1-800-633-4227) to find out if Medicare covers an item or service you need. TTY users should call 1-877-486-2048. If you're in a Medicare health plan, contact your plan.

If you have a question or complaint about the quality of a Medicare-covered service, call your Beneficiary and Family Centered Care Quality Improvement Organization (BFCC-QIO). Visit Medicare.gov/contacts to get your BFCC-QIO's phone number. You can also call 1-800-MEDICARE.

Paying for long-term care

Long-term care includes non-medical care for people who have a chronic illness or disability. This includes non-skilled personal care assistance, like help with everyday activities, including dressing, bathing, and using the bathroom. At least 70% of people over 65 will need long-term care services and support at some point. **Medicare and most health insurance plans, including Medicare Supplement Insurance (Medigap) policies, don't pay for this type of care, sometimes called "custodial care."** Long-term care can be provided at home, in the community, in an assisted living facility, or in a nursing home. It's important to start planning for long-term care now to maintain your independence and to make sure you get the care you may need, in the setting you want, in the future.

Here are some of the different ways to pay for long-term care:

Long-term care insurance—This type of private insurance can help pay for many types of long-term care, including both skilled and non-skilled (custodial) care. Long-term care insurance policies can vary widely. Some policies may cover only nursing home care. Others may include coverage for a range of services, like adult day care, assisted living, medical equipment, and informal home care.

Note: Long-term care insurance doesn't replace your Medicare coverage.

Your current or former employer or union may offer long-term care insurance. Current and retired federal employees, active and retired members of the uniformed services, and their qualified relatives can apply for coverage under the Federal Long-Term Care Insurance Program. If you have questions, visit opm.gov/insure/ltc, or call the Federal Long-Term Care Insurance Program at 1-800-582-3337. TTY users should call 1-800-843-3557.

Personal resources—Many people choose to use their own resources to pay for long-term care. Keep in mind that long-term care can be very expensive. It's important to know the financial risks before you decide to try to save enough money on your own. You should discuss your specific situation with your family members and a financial professional.

Other private options—Besides long-term care insurance and personal resources, some insurance companies let you use your life insurance policy to pay for long-term care. Ask your insurance agent how this works. Also, you may choose to pay for long-term care through a trust or annuity. The best option for you depends on your age, health status, risk of needing long-term care, and your personal financial situation. Visit longtermcare.gov for more information about your options.

Medicaid—Medicaid is a joint federal and state program that helps pay for certain health services for people with limited income and resources. If you qualify, you may be able to get help to pay for nursing home care or other health care costs.

If you're eligible for Medicaid, you may be able to get Medicaid services that help you stay in your home instead of moving to a nursing home. For more information, contact your State Medical Assistance (Medicaid) office. Visit Medicare.gov/contacts, or call 1-800-MEDICARE (1-800-633-4227) and say "Medicaid" to get the phone number. TTY users should call 1-877-486-2048. See pages 116–117 for more information about Medicaid.

Veterans' benefits—The Department of Veterans Affairs (VA) may provide long-term care for service-related disabilities or for certain eligible veterans. The VA also has a Housebound and Aid and Attendance Allowance Program that provides cash grants to eligible disabled veterans and surviving spouses. For more information, visit va.gov, or call the VA at 1-800-827-1000. TTY users should call 1-800-829-4833.

Definitions of blue words are on pages 145–148.

Programs of All-inclusive Care for the Elderly (PACE)—PACE is a Medicare and Medicaid program offered in many states that allows people who otherwise need a nursing home-level of care to remain in the community. See page 89 for more information.

What's the Long-Term Care Ombudsman?

Residents of long-term care facilities (like nursing homes, assisted living,

and board and care homes) also have access to a Long-Term Care Ombudsman. These ombudsmen provide information about how to find a facility, how to get quality care and can help you with complaints.

The Long-Term Care Ombudsman is funded by the Older Americans Act and is available to any long-term care facility resident. For more information, visit ltcombudsman.org. You can also call the Eldercare Locator at 1-800-677-1116 to get the phone number for your local ombudsman program office.

Long-term care contacts

Use these resources to get more information about long-term care:
- Visit longtermcare.gov to learn more about planning for long-term care.
- Visit Medicare.gov/nhcompare to compare nursing homes or Medicare.gov/homehealthcompare to compare home health agencies in your area.
- Call 1-800-MEDICARE (1-800-633-4227). TTY users should call 1-877-486-2048.
- Call your State Insurance Department to get information about long-term care insurance. Visit Medicare.gov/contacts, or call 1-800-MEDICARE to get the phone number.
- Call your State Health Insurance Assistance Program (SHIP). See pages 141–144 for the phone number.
- Call the National Association of Insurance Commissioners at 1-866-470-6242 to get a copy of "A Shopper's Guide to Long-Term Care Insurance."
- Visit the Eldercare Locator, a public service of the U.S. Administration on Aging, at eldercare.gov to find your local Aging and Disability Resource Center (ADRC). You can also call 1-800-677-1116. ADRCs offer a full range of long-term care services and support in a single, coordinated program.

Notes

Section 4—

What's Original Medicare?

How does Original Medicare work?

Original Medicare is one of your health coverage choices as part of Medicare. You'll have Original Medicare unless you choose a Medicare Advantage Plan (like an HMO or PPO).

Original Medicare is coverage managed by the federal government. You generally have to pay a portion of the cost for each service covered by Original Medicare. See the next page for the general rules about how it works.

	Original Medicare
Can I get my health care from any doctor, other health care provider, or hospital?	In most cases, yes. You can go to any doctor, other health care provider, hospital, or other facility that's enrolled in Medicare and accepting Medicare patients.
Are prescription drugs covered?	With a few exceptions (see pages 38 and 54), most prescriptions aren't covered. You can add drug coverage by joining a Medicare Prescription Drug Plan (Part D). See pages 97–110.
Do I need to choose a primary care doctor?	No.
Do I have to get a referral to see a specialist?	In most cases, no, but the specialist must be enrolled in Medicare.
Should I get a supplemental policy?	You may already have employer or union coverage that may pay costs that Original Medicare doesn't. If not, you may want to buy a Medicare Supplement Insurance (Medigap) policy if you're eligible. See pages 91–96.
What else do I need to know about Original Medicare?	▪ You generally pay a set amount for your health care (deductible) before Medicare pays its share. Then, Medicare pays its share, and you pay your share (coinsurance/copayment) for covered services and supplies. There's no yearly limit for what you pay out-of-pocket. ▪ You usually pay a monthly premium for Part B. See pages 115–116 for information about help paying your Part B premium. ▪ You generally don't need to file Medicare claims. The law requires providers (like doctors, hospitals, skilled nursing facilities, and home health agencies) and suppliers to file your claims for the covered services and supplies you get.

What do I pay?

Your out-of-pocket costs in Original Medicare depend on:

- Whether you have Part A and/or Part B. Most people have both.
- Whether your doctor, other health care provider, or supplier accepts "assignment."
- The type of health care you need and how often you need it.
- Whether you choose to get services or supplies Medicare doesn't cover. If you do, you pay all costs unless you have other insurance that covers it.
- Whether you have other health insurance that works with Medicare.
- Whether you have Medicaid or get help from your state paying your Medicare costs.
- Whether you have a Medicare Supplement Insurance (Medigap) policy.
- Whether you and your doctor or other health care provider sign a private contract. See page 72.

For more information on how other insurance works with Medicare, see pages 28–29. For more information about help to cover the costs that Original Medicare doesn't cover, see pages 115–116.

How do I know what Medicare paid?

If you have Original Medicare, you'll get a "Medicare Summary Notice" in the mail every 3 months that lists all the services billed to Medicare. The notice shows what Medicare paid and what you may owe the provider. This notice isn't a bill. Read it carefully and do this:

- If you have other insurance, check to see if it covers anything that Medicare didn't.
- Keep your receipts and bills, and compare them to your notice to be sure you got all the services, supplies, or equipment listed. See pages 128–131 for information on Medicare fraud.
- If you paid a bill before you got your notice, compare your notice with the bill to make sure you paid the right amount for your services.
- If an item or service is denied, call your doctor's or other health care provider's office to make sure they submitted the correct information. If not, the office may resubmit the claim.

If you disagree with any decision made, you can file an appeal. See pages 120–123.

Definitions of blue words are on pages 145–148.

If you need to change your address on your notice, call Social Security at 1-800-772-1213. TTY users should call 1-800-325-0778. If you get Railroad Retirement Board (RRB) benefits, call the RRB at 1-877-772-5772. TTY users should call 1-312-751-4701.

Important!

Check your claims on MyMedicare.gov

You don't have to wait for your Medicare Summary Notices to come in the mail to view your Medicare claims or file an appeal. Visit MyMedicare.gov to look at your Medicare claims or view electronic copies of your Medicare Summary Notices. Your claims generally will be available for viewing within 24 hours after processing. You can also download your claims information by using Medicare's Blue Button. See page 136.

What's assignment?

Assignment means that your doctor, provider, or supplier agrees (or is required by law) to accept the Medicare-approved amount as full payment for covered services.

Make sure your doctor, provider, or supplier accepts assignment

Most doctors, providers, and suppliers accept assignment, but you should always check to make sure. Participating providers have signed an agreement to accept assignment for all Medicare-covered services.

Important!

To find out if your doctors and other health care providers accept assignment or participate in Medicare, visit Medicare.gov/physician or Medicare.gov/supplier. You can also call 1-800-MEDICARE, or ask your doctor, provider, or supplier if they accept assignment.

Here's what happens if your doctor, provider, or supplier accepts assignment:

- Your out-of-pocket costs may be less.
- They agree to charge you only the Medicare deductible and coinsurance amount and usually wait for Medicare to pay its share before asking you to pay your share.
- They have to submit your claim directly to Medicare and can't charge you for submitting the claim.

Definitions of blue words are on pages 145–148.

If your doctor, provider, or supplier doesn't accept assignment

Non-participating providers haven't signed an agreement to accept assignment for all Medicare-covered services, but they can still choose to accept assignment for individual services. These providers are called "non-participating." Here's what happens if your doctor, provider, or supplier doesn't accept assignment:

- **You might have to pay the entire charge at the time of service.** Your doctor, provider, or supplier is supposed to submit a claim to Medicare for any Medicare-covered services they provide to you. They can't charge you for submitting a claim. If they don't submit the Medicare claim once you ask them to, call 1-800-MEDICARE (1-800-633-4227). TTY users should call 1-877-486-2048.

  Note: In some cases, you might have to submit your own claim to Medicare using form CMS-1490S to get paid back. Visit Medicare.gov/medicareonlineforms, or call 1-800-MEDICARE for the form and instructions.

- **They can charge you more than the Medicare-approved amount, but there's a limit called "the limiting charge."** The limiting charge applies only to certain Medicare-covered services and doesn't apply to some supplies and durable medical equipment. Call 1-800-MEDICARE to find out if you were charged the right amount.

What are private contracts?

A "private contract" is a written agreement between you and a doctor or other health care provider who has decided **not** to provide services to anyone through Medicare. The private contract only applies to the services provided by the doctor or other provider who asked you to sign it.

Rules for private contracts

You don't have to sign a private contract. You can always go to another provider who gives services through Medicare. If you sign a private contract with your doctor or other provider:

- **Medicare won't pay any amount for the services you get from this doctor or provider, even if it's a Medicare-covered service.**
- You'll have to pay the full amount of whatever this provider charges you for the services you get.
- If you have a Medicare Supplement Insurance (Medigap) policy, it won't pay anything for the services you get. Call your insurance company before you get the service if you have questions.
- Your provider must tell you if Medicare would pay for the service if you get it from another provider who accepts Medicare.
- Your provider must tell you if he or she has been excluded from Medicare.
- You can always get services not covered by Medicare if you choose to pay for them yourself.

Note: You can't be asked to sign a private contract for emergency or urgent care.

You should contact your State Health Insurance Assistance Program (SHIP) to get help before signing a private contract with any doctor or other health care provider. See pages 141–144 for the phone number.

Can I add drug coverage (Part D) to Original Medicare?

In Original Medicare, **if you don't already have** creditable prescription drug coverage (for example, from a current or former employer or union) and you would like Medicare prescription drug coverage, you must join a Medicare Prescription Drug Plan. These plans are available through private companies

under contract with Medicare. If you don't currently have creditable prescription drug coverage, you should think about joining a Medicare Prescription Drug Plan as soon as you're eligible. **If you don't have creditable prescription drug coverage and don't join a Medicare Prescription Drug Plan when you're first eligible, you may have to pay a late enrollment penalty if you decide to join later.** See pages 104–105 for more information.

If you have creditable prescription drug coverage from an employer or union, call your employer or union's benefits administrator before you make any changes to your coverage. Your employer or union plan will tell you each year if your prescription drug coverage is creditable. If you drop your employer or union coverage, you may not be able to get it back. You also may not be able to drop your employer or union **drug** coverage without also dropping your employer or union **health** (doctor and hospital) coverage. If you drop coverage for yourself, you may also have to drop coverage for your spouse and dependents.

Definitions of blue words are on pages 145–148.

Notes

Section 5—

Learn about Medicare Advantage Plans (Part C) & Other Medicare Health Plans

What are Medicare Advantage Plans?

A Medicare Advantage Plan (like an HMO or PPO) is another way to get your Medicare coverage. If you join a Medicare Advantage Plan, you still have Medicare. You'll get your Medicare Part A (Hospital Insurance) and Medicare Part B (Medical Insurance) coverage from the Medicare Advantage Plan, not Original Medicare. Medicare Advantage Plans, sometimes called "Part C" or "MA Plans," are offered by private companies that Medicare approves.

Medicare Advantage Plans cover all Medicare services

In all types of Medicare Advantage Plans, you're always covered for emergency and urgent care. Medicare Advantage Plans must cover all of the services that Original Medicare covers except hospice care and some care in qualifying clinical research studies. Original Medicare covers hospice care and some costs for clinical research studies, even if you're in a Medicare Advantage Plan.

Medicare Advantage Plans may offer extra coverage, like vision, hearing, dental, and other health and wellness programs. Most include Medicare prescription drug coverage (Part D). In addition to your Part B premium, you might pay a monthly premium for the Medicare Advantage Plan.

Definitions of blue words are on pages 145–148.

Medicare Advantage Plans must follow Medicare's rules

Medicare pays a fixed amount for your coverage each month to the companies offering Medicare Advantage Plans. These companies must follow rules set by Medicare. However, each Medicare Advantage Plan can charge different out-of-pocket costs and have different rules for how you get services (like whether you need a referral to see a specialist or if you have to go to doctors, facilities, or suppliers that belong to the plan's network for non-emergency or non-urgent care). These rules can change each year. The plan must notify you about any changes before the start of the next enrollment year.

Important!

Read the information you get from your plan

If you're in a Medicare Advantage Plan, review the "Evidence of Coverage" (EOC) and "Annual Notice of Change" (ANOC) your plan sends you each year. The EOC gives you details about what the plan covers, how much you pay, and more. The ANOC includes any changes in coverage, costs, provider networks, service area, and more that will be effective in January. If you don't get these important documents, contact your plan.

What are the different types of Medicare Advantage Plans?

- **Health Maintenance Organization (HMO) plans**—In most HMOs, you can only go to doctors, other health care providers, or hospitals in the plan's network except in an urgent or emergency situation. You may also need to get a referral from your primary care doctor for tests or to see other doctors or specialists. See page 82.
- **Preferred Provider Organization (PPO) plans**—In a PPO, you pay less if you use doctors, hospitals, and other health care providers that belong to the plan's network. You usually pay more if you use doctors, hospitals, and providers outside of the network. See page 83.
- **Private Fee-for-Service (PFFS) plans**—PFFS plans are similar to Original Medicare in that you can generally go to any doctor, other health care provider, or hospital as long as they agree to treat you. The plan determines how much it will pay doctors, other health care providers, and hospitals, and how much you must pay when you get care. See page 84.
- **Special Needs Plans (SNPs)**—SNPs provide focused and specialized health care for specific groups of people, like those who have both Medicare and Medicaid, live in a nursing home, or have certain chronic medical conditions. See page 85.

- **HMO Point-of-Service (HMOPOS) plans**—These are HMO plans that may allow you to get some services out-of-network for a higher copayment or coinsurance.
- **Medical Savings Account (MSA) plans**—These plans combine a high-deductible health plan with a bank account. Medicare deposits money into the account (usually less than the deductible). You can use the money to pay for your health care services during the year. MSA plans don't offer Medicare drug coverage. If you want drug coverage, you have to join a Medicare Prescription Drug Plan. For more information about MSAs, visit Medicare.gov/publications to view the booklet "Your Guide to Medicare Medical Savings Account Plans." You can also call 1-800-MEDICARE (1-800-633-4227) to find out if a copy can be mailed to you. TTY users should call 1-877-486-2048.

Important! Make sure you understand how a plan works before you join. See pages 82–86 for more information about Medicare Advantage Plan types. If you want more information about a Medicare Advantage Plan, you can call any plan and request a "Summary of Benefits" (SB) document. Contact your State Health Insurance Assistance Program (SHIP) for help comparing plans. See pages 141–144 for the phone number.

What else should I know about Medicare Advantage Plans?

- You have Medicare rights and protections, including the right to appeal. See pages 120–123.
- You can check with the plan before you get a service to find out if it's covered and what your costs may be.
- You must follow plan rules. It's important to check with the plan for information about your rights and responsibilities.
- If you go to a doctor, other health care provider, facility, or supplier that doesn't belong to the plan's network, your services may not be covered, or your costs could be higher. In most cases, this applies to Medicare Advantage HMOs and PPOs.
- Providers can join or leave a plan's provider network anytime during the year. Your plan can also change the providers in the network anytime during the year. If this happens, you may need to choose a new provider.

Definitions of blue words are on pages 145–148.

Definitions of blue words are on pages 145–148.

- If you join a clinical research study, some costs may be covered by Original Medicare and some may be covered by your Medicare Advantage Plan.
- Medicare Advantage Plans can't charge more than Original Medicare for certain services, like chemotherapy, dialysis, and skilled nursing facility care.
- Medicare Advantage Plans have a yearly limit on your out-of-pocket costs for medical services. Once you reach this limit, you'll pay nothing for covered services. This limit may be different between Medicare Advantage Plans and can change each year. You should consider this when choosing a plan.

Joining and leaving

- You can join a Medicare Advantage Plan even if you have a pre-existing condition, except for End-Stage Renal Disease (ESRD). See page 80.
- **You can only join or leave a Medicare Advantage Plan at certain times during the year.** See pages 86–87.
- Each year, Medicare Advantage Plans can choose to leave Medicare or make changes to the services they cover and what you pay. If the plan decides to stop participating in Medicare, you'll have to join another Medicare Advantage Plan or return to Original Medicare. See page 120.
- Medicare Advantage Plans must follow certain rules when giving you information about how to join their plan. See page 130 for more information about these rules and how to protect your personal information.

Prescription drug coverage

You usually get prescription drug coverage (Part D) through the Medicare Advantage Plan. In certain types of Medicare Advantage Plans (PFFS or MSA plans) that don't offer drug coverage, you can join a Medicare Prescription Drug Plan. **If your Medicare Advantage Plan includes prescription drug coverage and you join a Medicare Prescription Drug Plan, you'll be disenrolled from your Medicare Advantage Plan and returned to Original Medicare.**

Who can join?

You must meet these conditions to join a Medicare Advantage Plan:

- You have Part A and Part B.
- You live in the plan's service area.
- You don't have End-Stage Renal Disease (ESRD), except as explained on page 80.

What if I have other coverage?

Talk to your employer, union, or other benefits administrator about their rules before you join a Medicare Advantage Plan. In some cases, joining a Medicare Advantage Plan might cause you to lose your employer or union coverage. If you lose coverage for yourself, you may also lose coverage for your spouse and dependents. In other cases, if you join a Medicare Advantage Plan, you may still be able to use your employer or union coverage along with the plan you join. **Remember, if you drop your employer or union coverage, you may not be able to get it back.**

What if I have a Medicare Supplement Insurance (Medigap) Policy?

You can't use (and can't be sold) a Medicare Supplement Insurance (Medigap) policy while you're in a Medicare Advantage Plan.

You can't use it to pay for any expenses (copayments, deductibles, and premiums) you have under a Medicare Advantage Plan. If you already have a Medigap policy and join a Medicare Advantage Plan, you'll probably want to drop your Medigap policy. **If you drop your Medigap policy, you may not be able to get it back.** See page 95.

What if I have End-Stage Renal Disease (ESRD)?

If you have End-Stage Renal Disease (ESRD), you can only join a Medicare Advantage Plan in certain situations:

- If you're already in a Medicare Advantage Plan when you develop ESRD, you can stay in your plan or you may be able to join another Medicare Advantage Plan offered by the same company.
- If you're in a Medicare Advantage Plan, and the plan leaves Medicare or no longer provides coverage in your area, you have a one-time right to join another Medicare Advantage Plan.
- If you have an employer or union health plan or other health coverage through a company that offers one or more Medicare Advantage Plan(s), you may be able to join one of that company's Medicare Advantage Plans.
- If you've had a successful kidney transplant, you may be able to join a Medicare Advantage Plan.
- You may be able to join a Medicare Special Needs Plan (SNP) that covers people with ESRD if one is available in your area.

For more information visit Medicare.gov/publications to view the booklet "Medicare Coverage of Kidney Dialysis & Kidney Transplant Services." You can also call 1-800-MEDICARE (1-800-633-4227) to find out if a copy can be mailed to you. TTY users should call 1-877-486-2048.

Note: If you have ESRD and Original Medicare, you may join a Medicare Prescription Drug Plan.

Definitions of blue words are on pages 145–148.

What do I pay?

Your out-of-pocket costs in a Medicare Advantage Plan depend on:

- Whether the plan charges a monthly premium in addition to your monthly Part B premium.
- Whether the plan pays any of your monthly Part B premium.
- Whether the plan has a yearly deductible or any additional deductibles for certain services.
- How much you pay for each visit or service (copayments or coinsurance).
- The type of health care services you need and how often you get them.
- Whether you go to a doctor or supplier who accepts assignment (if you're in a Preferred Provider Organization, Private Fee-for-Service Plan, or Medical Savings Account Plan and you go out-of-network). See pages 70–71 for more information about assignment.
- Whether you follow the plan's rules, like using network providers.
- Whether you need extra benefits and if the plan charges for them.
- The plan's yearly limit on your out-of-pocket costs for all medical services. Once you reach this limit, you'll pay nothing for covered services.
- Whether you have Medicaid or get help from your state.

To learn more about your costs in specific Medicare Advantage Plans, visit Medicare.gov/find-a-plan. You can also call 1-800-MEDICARE (1-800-633-4227). TTY users should call 1-877-486-2048.

HMO

Types of Medicare Advantage Plans

Health Maintenance Organization (HMO) plan

Can I get my health care from any doctor, other health care provider, or hospital?

No. You generally must get your care and services from doctors, other health care providers, or hospitals in the plan's network (except emergency care, out-of-area urgent care, or out-of-area dialysis). In some plans, you may be able to go out-of-network for certain services, usually for a higher cost. This is called an HMO with a point-of-service (POS) option.

Are prescription drugs covered?

In most cases, yes. Ask the plan. If you want Medicare drug coverage, you must join an HMO plan that offers prescription drug coverage.

Do I need to choose a primary care doctor?

In most cases, yes.

Do I have to get a referral to see a specialist?

In most cases, yes. Certain services, like yearly screening mammograms, don't require a referral.

What else do I need to know about this type of plan?

- If your doctor or other health care provider leaves the plan, your plan will notify you. You can choose another doctor in the plan.
- If you get health care outside the plan's network, you may have to pay the full cost.
- It's important that you follow the plan's rules, like getting prior approval for a certain service when needed.

Definitions of blue words are on pages 145–148.

Preferred Provider Organization (PPO) plan

Can I get my health care from any doctor, other health care provider, or hospital?

In most cases, yes. PPOs have network doctors, other health care providers, and hospitals, but you can also use out-of-network providers for covered services, usually for a higher cost.

Are prescription drugs covered?

In most cases, yes. Ask the plan. If you want Medicare drug coverage, you must join a PPO plan that offers prescription drug coverage.

Do I need to choose a primary care doctor?

No.

Do I have to get a referral to see a specialist?

In most cases, no.

What else do I need to know about this type of plan?

- PPO plans aren't the same as Original Medicare or Medigap.
- Medicare PPO plans usually offer more benefits than Original Medicare, but you may have to pay extra for these benefits.

PFFS

Private Fee-for-Service (PFFS) plan

Can I get my health care from any doctor, other health care provider, or hospital?

In some cases, yes. You can go to any Medicare-approved doctor, other health care provider, or hospital that accepts the plan's payment terms and agrees to treat you. Not all providers will. If you join a PFFS plan that has a network, you can also see any of the network providers who have agreed to always treat plan members. You can also choose an out-of-network doctor, hospital, or other provider, who accepts the plan's terms, but you may pay more.

Are prescription drugs covered?

Sometimes. If your PFFS plan doesn't offer drug coverage, you can join a Medicare Prescription Drug Plan (Part D) to get coverage.

Do I need to choose a primary care doctor?

No.

Do I have to get a referral to see a specialist?

No.

What else do I need to know about this type of plan?

- PFFS plans aren't the same as Original Medicare or Medigap.
- The plan decides how much you must pay for services.
- Some PFFS plans contract with a network of providers who agree to always treat you even if you've never seen them before.
- Out-of-network doctors, hospitals, and other providers may decide not to treat you even if you've seen them before.
- For each service you get, make sure your doctors, hospitals, and other providers agree to treat you under the plan, and accept the plan's payment terms.
- In an emergency, doctors, hospitals, and other providers must treat you.

Definitions of blue words are on pages 145–148.

Special Needs Plan (SNP)

Can I get my health care from any doctor, other health care provider, or hospital?

You generally must get your care and services from doctors, other health care providers, or hospitals in the plan's network (except emergency care, out-of-area urgent care, or out-of-area dialysis).

Are prescription drugs covered?

Yes. All SNPs must provide Medicare prescription drug coverage (Part D).

Do I need to choose a primary care doctor?

Generally, yes.

Do I have to get a referral to see a specialist?

In most cases, yes. Certain services, like yearly screening mammograms, don't require a referral.

What else do I need to know about this type of plan?

- A plan must limit membership to these groups: 1) people who live in certain institutions (like nursing homes) or who require nursing care at home, or 2) people who are eligible for both Medicare and Medicaid, or 3) people who have specific chronic or disabling conditions (like diabetes, ESRD, HIV/AIDS, chronic heart failure, or dementia). Plans may further limit membership.

- Plans should coordinate the services and providers you need to help you stay healthy and follow doctor's or other health care provider's orders.

- For more information about SNPs, visit Medicare.gov/publications to view the booklet "Your Guide to Medicare Special Needs Plans (SNPs)."

When can I join, switch, or drop a Medicare Advantage Plan?

- **When you first become eligible for Medicare,** you can join during the 7-month period that begins 3 months before the month you turn 65, includes the month you turn 65, and ends 3 months after the month you turn 65.
- **If you get Medicare due to a disability,** you can join during the 7-month period that begins 3 months before your 25th month of disability and ends 3 months after your 25th month of disability.
- **Between October 15–December 7 anyone with Medicare can join, switch, or drop a Medicare Advantage Plan.** Your coverage will begin on January 1, as long as the plan gets your request by December 7.

Can I make changes to my coverage after December 7?

Between January 1–February 14, if you're in a Medicare Advantage Plan, you can leave that plan and switch to Original Medicare. If you switch to Original Medicare during this period, you'll have until February 14 to also join a Medicare Prescription Drug Plan to add drug coverage. Your coverage will begin the first day of the month after the plan gets your enrollment request. During this period, you **can't:**

- Switch from Original Medicare to a Medicare Advantage Plan.
- Switch from one Medicare Advantage Plan to another.
- Switch from one Medicare Prescription Drug Plan to another.
- Join, switch, or drop a Medicare Medical Savings Account Plan.

Special Enrollment Periods

In most cases, you must stay enrolled for the calendar year starting the date your coverage begins. However, in certain situations, you may be able to join, switch, or drop a Medicare Advantage Plan during a Special Enrollment Period. Some examples are:

- You move out of your plan's service area.
- You have Medicaid.
- You qualify for Extra Help. See pages 111–115.
- You live in an institution (like a nursing home).

Definitions of blue words are on pages 145–148.

5-Star Special Enrollment Period

Medicare uses information on plan performance including how good the care is and the results of care, as well as surveys from members to rate the overall performance of Medicare Advantage Plans. A Medicare Advantage Plan can get an overall rating between 1 and 5 stars. A 5-star rating is considered excellent. These ratings help you compare Medicare Advantage Plans based on quality and performance. These ratings are updated each fall and can change each year.

You can switch to a Medicare Advantage Plan or Medicare Cost Plan (see page 88) that has **5 stars for its overall star rating** from December 8, 2014–November 30, 2015.

- The overall star ratings are available at Medicare.gov/find-a-plan.
- You can only join a 5-star Medicare Advantage Plan or Medicare Cost Plan if one is available in your area.
- You can only use this Special Enrollment Period once during the above timeframe.

For more information about overall star ratings, visit Medicare.gov.

Important! You may lose your prescription drug coverage if you move from a Medicare Advantage Plan that has drug coverage to a 5-star Medicare Advantage Plan that doesn't. You'll have to wait until the next Open Enrollment Period to get drug coverage, and you may have to pay a late enrollment penalty. See pages 104–105.

How do I switch?

Follow these steps if you're already in a Medicare Advantage Plan and want to switch:

- **To switch to a new Medicare Advantage Plan,** simply join the plan you choose during one of the enrollment periods explained on pages 86–87. You'll be disenrolled automatically from your old plan when your new plan's coverage begins.
- **To switch to Original Medicare,** contact your current plan, or call 1-800-MEDICARE (1-800-633-4227). TTY users should call 1-877-486-2048. If you don't have drug coverage, you should carefully consider joining a Medicare Prescription Drug Plan. You may also want to consider a Medicare Supplement Insurance (Medigap) policy if you're eligible. See page 94 for more information about buying a Medigap policy.

For more information on joining, dropping, and switching plans, visit Medicare.gov/publications to view the fact sheet "Understanding Medicare Part C & D Enrollment Periods." You can also call 1-800-MEDICARE (1-800-633-4227), to find out if a copy can be mailed to you. TTY users should call 1-877-486-2048.

Are there other types of Medicare health plans?

Some types of Medicare health plans that provide health care coverage aren't Medicare Advantage Plans but are still part of Medicare. Some of these plans provide Medicare Part A (Hospital Insurance) and Medicare Part B (Medical Insurance) coverage, while most others provide only Part B coverage. In addition, some also provide Part D prescription drug coverage. These plans have some of the same rules as Medicare Advantage Plans. However, each type of plan has special rules and exceptions, so you should contact any plans you're interested in to get more details.

Medicare Cost Plans

Medicare Cost Plans are a type of Medicare health plan available in certain areas of the country. Here's what you should know about Medicare Cost Plans:

- You can join even if you only have Part B.
- If you have Part A and Part B and go to a non-network provider, the services are covered under Original Medicare. You would pay the Part A and Part B coinsurance and deductibles.
- You can join anytime the Cost Plan is accepting new members.
- You can leave anytime and return to Original Medicare.
- You can either get your Medicare prescription drug coverage from the Cost Plan (if offered), or you can join a Medicare Prescription Drug Plan.

   Note: You can add or drop Medicare prescription drug coverage only at certain times. See pages 98–99.

Definitions of blue words are on pages 145–148.

There's another type of Medicare Cost Plan that only provides coverage for Part B services. These plans are either sponsored by employer or union group health plans, or offered by companies that don't provide Part A services. Part A services are covered through Original Medicare. These plans never include Part D.

For more information about Medicare Cost Plans, visit the Medicare Plan Finder at Medicare.gov/find-a-plan. Your State Health Insurance Assistance Program (SHIP) can also give you more information. See pages 141–144 for the phone number.

Programs of All-inclusive Care for the Elderly (PACE)

PACE is a Medicare and Medicaid program offered in many states that allows people who otherwise need a nursing home-level of care to remain in the community. To qualify for PACE, you must meet these conditions:

- You're 55 or older.
- You live in the service area of a PACE organization.
- You're certified by your state as needing a nursing home-level of care.
- At the time you join, you're able to live safely in the community with the help of PACE services.

PACE provides coverage for many services, including prescription drugs, doctor or other health care practitioner visits, transportation, home care, hospital visits, and even nursing home stays whenever necessary.

If you have Medicaid, you won't have to pay a monthly premium for the long-term care portion of the PACE benefit. If you have Medicare but not Medicaid, you'll be charged a monthly premium to cover the long-term care portion of the PACE benefit and a premium for Medicare Part D drugs. However, in PACE, there's never a deductible or copayment for any drug, service, or care approved by the PACE team of health care professionals.

Visit pace4you.org, or call your State Medical Assistance (Medicaid) office to find out if you're eligible and if there's a PACE site near you.

Medicare Innovation Projects

Medicare develops innovative models, demonstrations, and pilot projects to test and measure the effect of potential changes in Medicare. These projects help to find new ways to improve health care quality and reduce costs. Usually, they operate only for a limited time for a specific group of people and/or are offered only in specific areas. Some examples that are explained in this handbook include certain

Accountable Care Organizations (see page 138), and demonstration plans for people who have both Medicare and Medicaid (see page 117). Check with the model, demonstration, or pilot project (or with your health care provider) for more information about how they work. To learn more about the current Medicare models, demonstrations, and pilot projects, visit innovation.cms.gov. You can also call 1-800-MEDICARE (1-800-633-4227). TTY users should call 1-877-486-2048.

Definitions of blue words are on pages 145–148.

Section 6—

What are Medicare Supplement Insurance (Medigap) Policies?

Original Medicare pays for many, but not all, health care services and supplies. Medicare Supplement Insurance policies, sold by private companies, can help pay some of the health care costs that Original Medicare doesn't cover, like copayments, coinsurance, and deductibles. **Medicare Supplement Insurance policies are also called Medigap policies.**

Some Medigap policies also offer coverage for services that Original Medicare doesn't cover, like medical care when you travel outside the U.S. If you have Original Medicare and you buy a Medigap policy, Medicare will pay its share of the Medicare-approved amount for covered health care costs. Then, your Medigap policy pays its share. You have to pay the premiums for a Medigap policy.

Medigap policies are standardized

Every Medigap policy must follow federal and state laws designed to protect you, and it must be clearly identified as "Medicare Supplement Insurance." Insurance companies can sell you only a "standardized" policy identified in most states by letters A through D, F through G, and K through N. All policies offer the same basic benefits, but some offer additional benefits so you can choose which one meets your needs. In Massachusetts, Minnesota, and Wisconsin, Medigap policies are standardized in a different way.

Note: Plans E, H, I, and J are no longer available to buy, but if you already have one of those policies, you can keep it. Contact your insurance company for more information.

How do I compare Medigap policies?

Different insurance companies may charge different premiums for the same exact policy. As you shop for a policy, be sure you're comparing the same policy (for example, compare Plan A from one company with Plan A from another company).

In some states, you may be able to buy a type of Medigap policy called Medicare SELECT (a policy that requires you to use specific hospitals and, in some cases, specific doctors or other health care providers to get full coverage). If you buy a Medicare SELECT policy, you have the right to change your mind within 12 months and switch to a standard Medigap policy.

Definitions of blue words are on pages 145–148.

The chart below shows basic information about the different benefits that Medigap policies cover. If a percentage appears, the Medigap plan covers that percentage of the benefit, and you're responsible for the rest.

Note: You'll need more details than this chart provides to compare and choose a policy. See page 96 to find out where to get more information.

Benefits	Medicare Supplement Insurance (Medigap) plans									
	A	**B**	**C**	**D**	**F***	**G**	**K**	**L**	**M**	**N**
Medicare Part A coinsurance and hospital costs (up to an additional 365 days after Medicare benefits are used)	100%	100%	100%	100%	100%	100%	100%	100%	100%	100%
Medicare Part B coinsurance or copayment	100%	100%	100%	100%	100%	100%	50%	75%	100%	100% **
Blood (first 3 pints)	100%	100%	100%	100%	100%	100%	50%	75%	100%	100%
Part A hospice care coinsurance or copayment	100%	100%	100%	100%	100%	100%	50%	75%	100%	100%
Skilled nursing facility care coinsurance			100%	100%	100%	100%	50%	75%	100%	100%
Part A deductible		100%	100%	100%	100%	100%	50%	75%	50%	100%
Part B deductible			100%		100%					
Part B excess charges					100%	100%				
Foreign travel emergency (up to plan limits)			80%	80%	80%	80%			80%	80%
							Out-of-pocket limit in 2014			
							$4,940	$2,470		

* Plan F also offers a high-deductible plan in some states. If you choose this option, this means you must pay for Medicare-covered costs (coinsurance, copayments, and deductibles) up to the deductible amount of $2,140 in 2014 before your policy pays anything.

** Plan N pays 100% of the Part B coinsurance, except for a copayment of up to $20 for some office visits and up to a $50 copayment for emergency room visits that don't result in an inpatient admission.

What else should I know about Medicare Supplement Insurance (Medigap)?

Important facts

- You must have Part A and Part B.
- You pay the private insurance company a monthly premium for your Medigap policy in addition to your monthly Part B premium that you pay to Medicare. Contact the company to find out how to pay your premium.
- A Medigap policy only covers one person. Spouses must buy separate policies.
- You can't have prescription drug coverage in both your Medigap policy and a Medicare drug plan. See page 109.
- It's important to compare Medigap policies since the costs can vary and may go up as you get older. Some states limit Medigap premium costs.

When to buy

- The best time to buy a Medigap policy is during your Medigap Open Enrollment Period. This 6-month period begins on the first day of the month in which you're 65 or older **and** enrolled in Part B. (Some states have additional Open Enrollment Periods.) After this enrollment period, your option to buy a Medigap policy may be limited and it may cost more.
- If you delay enrolling in Part B because you have group health coverage based on your (or your spouse's) current employment, your Medigap Open Enrollment Period won't start until you sign up for Part B.
- Federal law doesn't require insurance companies to sell Medigap policies to people under 65. If you're under 65, you might not be able to buy the Medigap policy you want, or any Medigap policy, until you turn 65. However, some states require Medigap insurance companies to sell Medigap policies to people under 65.

Definitions of blue words are on pages 145–148.

How does Medigap work with Medicare Advantage Plans?

- If you have a Medicare Advantage Plan, it's illegal for anyone to sell you a Medigap policy unless you're switching back to Original Medicare. If you want to switch to Original Medicare and buy a Medigap policy, find out what policies are available to you and contact your Medicare Advantage Plan to see if you're able to disenroll. You'll need to let the Medigap insurer know the date your plan coverage will end. If you don't intend to leave your Medicare Advantage Plan, and someone tries to sell you a Medigap policy, report it to your State Insurance Department.

- If you have a Medigap policy and join a Medicare Advantage Plan (like an HMO or PPO), you may want to drop your Medigap policy. Your Medigap policy **can't** be used to pay your Medicare Advantage Plan copayments, deductibles, and premiums. If you want to cancel your Medigap policy, contact your insurance company. In most cases, if you drop your Medigap policy to join a Medicare Advantage Plan, you won't be able to get it back.

- If you join a Medicare Advantage Plan for the first time, and you aren't happy with the plan, you'll have special rights to buy a Medigap policy if you return to Original Medicare within 12 months of joining.

  —If you had a Medigap policy before you joined, you may be able to get the same policy back if the company still sells it. If it isn't available, you can buy another Medigap policy.

  —If you joined a Medicare Advantage Plan when you were first eligible for Medicare, you can choose from any Medigap policy within the first year of joining.

  —The Medigap policy can no longer have prescription drug coverage even if you had it before, but you may be able to join a Medicare Prescription Drug Plan.

Where can I get more information about Medicare Supplement Insurance (Medigap)?

- Visit Medicare.gov to find policies in your area.
- Visit Medicare.gov/publications to view the booklet "Choosing a Medigap Policy: A Guide to Health Insurance for People with Medicare." You can also call 1-800-MEDICARE (1-800-633-4227) to find out if a copy can be mailed to you. TTY users should call 1-877-486-2048.
- Call your State Insurance Department. Visit Medicare.gov/contacts, or call 1-800-MEDICARE to get the phone number.
- Call your State Health Insurance Assistance Program (SHIP). See pages 141–144 for the phone number.

Definitions of blue words are on pages 145–148.

Section 7—

Get Information about Prescription Drug Coverage (Part D)

How does Medicare prescription drug coverage (Part D) work?

Medicare offers prescription drug coverage to everyone with Medicare. Even if you don't take many prescriptions now, you should consider joining a Medicare drug plan. If you decide not to join a Medicare drug plan when you're first eligible, and you don't have other creditable prescription drug coverage, or you don't get Extra Help, you'll likely pay a late enrollment penalty if you join a plan later. See pages 104–105. To get Medicare prescription drug coverage, you must join a plan run by an insurance company or other private company approved by Medicare. Each plan can vary in cost and specific drugs covered.

There are 2 ways to get Medicare prescription drug coverage:

1. **Medicare Prescription Drug Plans.** These plans (sometimes called "PDPs") add drug coverage to Original Medicare, some Medicare Cost Plans, some Medicare Private Fee-for-Service (PFFS) plans, and Medicare Medical Savings Account (MSA) plans.

2. **Medicare Advantage Plans (like HMOs or PPOs) or other Medicare health plans that offer Medicare prescription drug coverage.** You get all of your Part A, Part B, and prescription drug coverage (Part D), through these plans. Medicare Advantage Plans with prescription drug coverage are sometimes called "MA-PDs." Remember, you must have Part A and Part B to join a Medicare Advantage Plan, and not all of these plans offer drug coverage.

In either case, you must live in the service area of the Medicare drug plan you want to join. **Both types of plans are called "Medicare drug plans" in this handbook.**

> **Important!**

If you have employer or union coverage

Call your benefits administrator before you make any changes, or before you sign up for any other coverage. If you drop your employer or union coverage, you may not be able to get it back. You also may not be able to drop your employer or union **drug** coverage without also dropping your employer or union **health** (doctor and hospital) coverage. If you drop coverage for yourself, you may also have to drop coverage for your spouse and dependents. If you want to know how Medicare prescription drug coverage works with other drug coverage you may have, see pages 108–110.

When can I join, switch, or drop a Medicare drug plan?

- **During your 7-month Initial Enrollment Period, when you first become eligible for Medicare.** You can join a Medicare drug plan during the 7-month period that begins 3 months before the month you turn 65, includes the month you turn 65, and ends 3 months after the month you turn 65. Your coverage will begin the first day of the month after you ask to join a plan. If you join during one of the 3 months before you turn 65, your coverage will begin the first day of the month you turn 65.

- **During your 7-month period around your 25th month of disability.** If you get Medicare due to a disability, you can join during the 7-month period that begins 3 months before your 25th month of entitlement to disability payments, includes your 25th month, and ends 3 months after your 25th month of entitlement to disability payments. Your coverage will begin the first day of the month after you ask to join a plan. If you join during one of the 3 months before you first get Medicare, your coverage will begin the first day of your 25th month of entitlement.

- **During Open Enrollment, between October 15–December 7 each year.** Your coverage begins on January 1 of the following year, as long as the plan gets your request during Open Enrollment.

- **At any time if you qualify for Extra Help.** See pages 111–115.

> Definitions of blue words are on pages 145–148.

Special Enrollment Periods

You generally must stay enrolled for the calendar year. However, in certain situations, you may be able to join, switch, or drop Medicare drug plans at other times. Some examples are if you:

- Move out of your plan's service area.
- Lose other creditable prescription drug coverage.
- Live in an institution (like a nursing home).
- Have Medicaid.
- Qualify for Extra Help. See pages 111–115.

5-Star Special Enrollment Period

You can switch to a Medicare Prescription Drug Plan that has **5 stars for its overall star rating** between December 8, 2014–November 30, 2015. The overall star ratings are available at Medicare.gov/find-a-plan. These ratings are updated each fall and can change each year. See page 87 for more information.

- You can only switch to a 5-star Medicare Prescription Drug Plan if one is available in your area.
- You can only use this Special Enrollment Period once during the time noted above.

For more information about overall star ratings, visit Medicare.gov.

Important!

If you have a Medicare Advantage Plan

If your Medicare Advantage Plan includes prescription drug coverage and you join a Medicare Prescription Drug Plan, you'll be disenrolled from your Medicare Advantage Plan and returned to Original Medicare.

How do I switch?

You can switch to a new Medicare drug plan simply by joining another drug plan during one of the times listed on pages 98–99. **You don't need to cancel your old Medicare drug plan.** Your old Medicare drug plan coverage will end when your new drug plan begins. You should get a letter from your new Medicare drug plan telling you when your coverage with the new plan begins.

How do I drop a Medicare drug plan?

If you want to drop your Medicare drug plan and you don't want to join a new plan, you can only do so during certain

times. See pages 98–99. You can disenroll by calling 1-800-MEDICARE (1-800-633-4227). TTY users should call 1-877-486-2048. You can also send a letter to the plan to tell them you want to disenroll. If you drop your plan and want to join another Medicare drug plan later, you have to wait for an enrollment period. You may have to pay a late enrollment penalty. See pages 104–105.

How much do I pay?

Below and continued on the next page are descriptions of what you pay in your Medicare drug plan. **Your actual drug plan costs will vary depending on:**

- Your prescriptions and whether they're on your plan's formulary (drug list).
- The plan you choose.
- Which pharmacy you use (preferred, non-preferred, out-of-network, or mail order).
- Whether you get Extra Help paying your Part D costs. See pages 111–115.

Monthly premium

Most drug plans charge a monthly fee that varies by plan. You pay this in addition to the Part B premium. If you're in a Medicare Advantage Plan (like an HMO or PPO) or a Medicare Cost Plan that includes Medicare prescription drug coverage, the monthly premium may include an amount for prescription drug coverage.

Note: Contact your drug plan (not Social Security or the Railroad Retirement Board (RRB)) if you want your premium deducted from your monthly Social Security or RRB payment. If you want to stop premium deductions and get billed directly, contact your drug plan.

Definitions of blue words are on pages 145–148.

Important!

If you have a higher income, you might pay more for your Part D coverage. If your income is above a certain limit ($85,000 if you file individually or $170,000 if you're married and file jointly), you'll pay an extra amount in addition to your plan premium. This doesn't affect everyone, so most people won't have to pay a higher amount.

Usually, the extra amount will be deducted from your Social Security check. If you get benefits from the Railroad Retirement Board (RRB), the extra amount will be deducted from your RRB check starting in 2015. **If you're billed the amount by Medicare or the RRB, you must pay the extra amount to Medicare or the RRB and not your plan.** If you have to pay an extra amount and you disagree (for example, you have a life event that lowers your income), call Social Security at 1-800-772-1213. TTY users should call 1-800-325-0778. For more information, visit socialsecurity.gov/pubs/EN-05-10536.pdf to view the fact sheet "Medicare Premiums: Rules for Higher-Income Beneficiaries."

Yearly deductible

This is the amount you must pay before your drug plan begins to pay its share of your covered drugs. Some drug plans don't have a deductible.

Copayments or coinsurance

These are the amounts you pay for your covered prescriptions after the deductible (if the plan has one). You pay your share and your drug plan pays its share for covered drugs. These amounts may vary.

Coverage gap

Most Medicare drug plans have a coverage gap (also called the "donut hole"). The coverage gap begins after you and your drug plan together have spent a certain amount for covered drugs. In 2015, once you enter the coverage gap, you pay 45% of the plan's cost for covered brand-name drugs and 65% of the plan's cost for covered generic drugs until you reach the end of the coverage gap. Not everyone will enter the coverage gap because their drug costs won't be high enough.

These items all **count** toward you getting out of the coverage gap:

- Your yearly deductible, coinsurance, and copayments
- The discount you get on covered brand-name drugs in the coverage gap
- What you pay in the coverage gap

The drug plan premium and what you pay for drugs that aren't covered **don't count** toward getting you out of the coverage gap.

Some plans offer additional cost-sharing reductions in the gap beyond the standard benefits and discounts on brand-name and generic drugs, but they may charge a higher monthly premium. Check with the plan first to see if your drugs would have additional cost-sharing reductions during the gap.

In addition to the discount on covered brand-name prescription drugs, there will be increasing coverage for brand-name and generic drugs in the coverage gap each year until the gap closes in 2020.

Catastrophic coverage

Once you get out of the coverage gap, you automatically get "catastrophic coverage." With catastrophic coverage, you only pay a small coinsurance amount or copayment for covered drugs for the rest of the year.

Note: If you get Extra Help, you won't have some of these costs. See pages 111–115.

Important!

Usually, the amount you pay for a covered prescription is for a month's supply of a drug. However, you can request less than a month's supply for most types of drugs. Some examples of when you might do this would be if you're trying a new medication that's known to have significant side effects or you want to synchronize the refills for all your medications. In these cases, the amount you pay is reduced based on the day's supply you actually get. Talk with your prescriber, because he or she will need to write you a prescription for this smaller supply.

Definitions of blue words are on pages 145–148.

The example below shows costs for covered drugs in 2015 for a plan that has a coverage gap.

Ms. Smith joins the ABC Prescription Drug Plan. Her coverage begins on January 1, 2015. She doesn't get Extra Help and uses her Medicare drug plan membership card when she buys prescriptions.

Monthly premium—Ms. Smith pays a monthly premium throughout the year			
1. Yearly deductible	2. Copayment or coinsurance (what she pays at the pharmacy)	3. Coverage gap	4. Catastrophic coverage
Ms. Smith pays the first $320 of her drug costs before her plan starts to pay its share.	Ms. Smith pays a copayment, and her plan pays its share for each covered drug until their combined amount (plus the deductible) reaches $2,960.	Once Ms. Smith and her plan have spent $2,960 for covered drugs, she's in the coverage gap. In 2015, she pays 45% of the plan's cost for her covered brand-name prescription drugs and 65% of the plan's cost for covered generic drugs. What she pays (and the discount paid by the drug company) counts as out-of-pocket spending, and helps her get out of the coverage gap.	Once Ms. Smith has spent $4,700 out-of-pocket for the year, her coverage gap ends. Now she only pays a small coinsurance or copayment for each covered drug until the end of the year.

Important! Visit Medicare.gov/find-a-plan to compare the costs of plans in your area. You can also call 1-800-MEDICARE (1-800-633-4227). TTY users should call 1-877-486-2048. For help comparing plan costs, contact your State Health Insurance Assistance Program (SHIP). See pages 141–144 for the phone number.

What's the Part D enrollment penalty?

The late enrollment penalty is an amount that's added to your Part D premium. You may owe a late enrollment penalty if at any time after your Initial Enrollment Period is over, there's a period of 63 or more days in a row when you don't have Part D or other creditable prescription drug coverage.

Note: If you get Extra Help, you don't pay a late enrollment penalty.

3 ways to avoid paying a penalty:

1. **Join a Medicare drug plan when you're first eligible.** Even if you don't take many prescriptions now, you should consider joining a Medicare drug plan to avoid a penalty. You may be able to find a plan that meets your needs with little to no monthly premiums.

2. **Don't go 63 days or more in a row without a Medicare drug plan or other creditable coverage.** Creditable prescription drug coverage could include drug coverage from a current or former employer or union, TRICARE, Indian Health Services, the Department of Veterans Affairs, or health coverage. Your plan must tell you each year if your drug coverage is creditable coverage. This information may be sent to you in a letter or included in a newsletter from the plan. Keep this information, because you may need it if you join a Medicare drug plan later.

3. **Tell your plan about any drug coverage you had if they ask about it.** When you join a Medicare drug plan, and the plan believes you went at least 63 days in a row without other creditable prescription drug coverage, the plan will send you a letter. The letter will include a form asking about any drug coverage you had. Complete the form, and return it to your drug plan. If you don't tell the plan about your creditable prescription drug coverage, you may have to pay a penalty.

Definitions of blue words are on pages 145–148.

How much more will I pay?

The cost of the late enrollment penalty depends on how long you didn't have creditable prescription drug coverage. Currently, the late enrollment penalty is calculated by multiplying 1% of the "national base beneficiary premium" ($32.42 in 2014) by the number of full, uncovered months that you were eligible but didn't join a Medicare drug plan and went without other creditable prescription drug coverage. The final amount is rounded to the nearest $.10 and added to your monthly premium. Since the "national base beneficiary premium" may increase each year, the penalty amount may also increase each year. You may have to pay this penalty for as long as you have a Medicare drug plan. After you join a Medicare drug plan, the plan will tell you if you owe a penalty and what your premium will be.

Example:

Mrs. Martin didn't join when she was first eligible—by June 2011. She doesn't have prescription drug coverage from any other source. She joined a Medicare drug plan during the 2013 Open Enrollment Period, and her coverage began on January 1, 2014.

Since Mrs. Martin was without creditable prescription drug coverage from July 2011–December 2013, her penalty in 2014 is 30% (1% for each of the 30 months) of $32.42 (the national base beneficiary premium for 2014), which is $9.73. The monthly penalty is rounded to the nearest $.10, so she'll be charged $9.70 each month in addition to her plan's monthly premium in 2014.

Here's the math:

.30 (30% penalty) × **$32.42** (2014 base beneficiary premium) = **$9.73**

$9.73 (rounded to the nearest $0.10) = **$9.70**

$9.70 = Mrs. Martin's monthly late enrollment penalty for 2014

What if I don't agree with the penalty?

If you don't agree with your late enrollment penalty, you can ask for a review or reconsideration. You'll need to fill out a reconsideration request form (that your Medicare drug plan will send you), and you'll have the chance to provide proof that supports your case, like information about previous creditable prescription drug coverage.

If you need help, call your plan.

Which drugs are covered?

Information about a plan's list of covered drugs (called a "formulary") isn't included in this handbook because each plan has its own formulary. Many Medicare drug plans place drugs into different "tiers" on their formularies. Drugs in each tier have a different cost. For example, a drug in a lower tier will generally cost you less than a drug in a higher tier. In some cases, if your drug is in a higher tier and your prescriber (your doctor or other health care provider who is legally allowed to write prescriptions) thinks you need that drug instead of a similar drug in a lower tier, you or your prescriber can ask your plan for an exception to get a lower copayment for the drug in the higher tier.

Contact the plan for its current formulary, or visit the plan's website. You can also visit the Medicare Plan Finder at Medicare.gov/find-a-plan, or call 1-800-MEDICARE (1-800-633-4227). TTY users should call 1-877-486-2048. Your plan will notify you of any formulary changes.

Important!

Each month that you fill a prescription, your drug plan mails you an "Explanation of Benefits" (EOB) notice. This notice gives you a summary of your prescription drug claims and your costs. Review your notice and check it for mistakes. Contact your plan if you have questions or find mistakes. If you suspect fraud, call the Medicare Drug Integrity Contractor (MEDIC) at 1-877-7SAFERX (1-877-772-3379). See page 130 for more information about the MEDIC.

Plans may have these coverage rules:

- **Prior authorization**—You and/or your prescriber must contact the drug plan before you can fill certain prescriptions. Your prescriber may need to show that the drug is medically necessary for the plan to cover it.
- **Quantity limits**—Limits on how much medication you can get at a time.
- **Step therapy**—You must try one or more similar, lower cost drugs before the plan will cover the prescribed drug.

If you or your prescriber believe that one of these coverage rules should be waived, you can ask for an exception. See page 122.

Definitions of blue words are on pages 145–148.

Starting in mid-2015, your prescribers need to be enrolled in Medicare or have an "opt-out" request on file with Medicare for your prescriptions to be covered by your Medicare drug plan. Contact your plan or your prescribers for more information.

Do you get automatic prescription refills in the mail?

Some people with Medicare get their prescription drugs by using an "automatic refill" service that automatically delivers prescription drugs when you're about to run out. To make sure you still need a prescription before they send you a refill, prescription drug plans should get your approval to deliver a new or refilled prescription before each delivery, except when you ask for the refill or new prescription. Be sure to give your drug plan the best way to reach you so you don't miss the refill confirmation call or other communication. The plan won't automatically ship your refills unless you confirm you still want to get the order. If you get a prescription automatically by mail that you don't want, and you weren't contacted to see if you wanted it before it shipped, you may be eligible for a refund. Did you know you can also sign up online for automatic refills with some pharmacies or get your prescription history? Visit bluebuttonconnector.healthit.gov to learn how.

Medication Therapy Management (MTM) Program

If you're in a Medicare drug plan and take medications for different medical conditions, you may be eligible to get services, at no cost to you, through a MTM program. This program helps you and your doctor make sure that your medications are working to improve your health. A pharmacist or other health professional will give you a comprehensive review of all your medications and talk with you about:

- How to get the most benefit from the drugs you take
- Any concerns you have, like medication costs and drug reactions
- How best to take your medications
- Any questions or problems you have about your prescription and over-the-counter medication

You'll get a written summary of this discussion. The summary has a medication action plan that recommends what you can do to make the best use of your medications, with space for you to take notes or write down any follow-up questions. You'll also get a personal medication list that will include all the medications you're taking and why you take them. Have this summary available when you talk with your health care providers.

It's a good idea to schedule your medication review before your yearly "Wellness" visit, so you can talk to your doctor about your action plan and medication list. Bring your action plan and medication list with you to your visit or anytime you talk with your doctors, pharmacists, and other health care providers. Also, take your medication list with you if you go to the hospital or emergency room.

Your drug plan may enroll you in this program if you meet all of these conditions:

1. You have more than one chronic health condition.

2. You take several different medications.

3. Your medications have a combined cost of more than $3,138 per year. This dollar amount (which can change each year) is estimated based on your out-of-pocket costs and the costs your plan pays for the medications each calendar year. Your plan can help you find out if you may reach this dollar limit.

Visit Medicare.gov/find-a-plan to get general information about program eligibility for your Medicare drug plan or for other plans that interest you. Contact each drug plan for specific details.

How do other insurance and programs work with Part D?

The charts on this page and the next 2 pages provide information about how other insurance you have works with, or is affected by, Medicare prescription drug coverage (Part D).

Employer or union health coverage—Health coverage from your, your spouse's, or other family member's current or former employer or union. If you have prescription drug coverage based on your current or previous employment, your employer or union will notify you each year to let you know if your prescription drug coverage is creditable. **Keep the information you get.** Call your benefits administrator for more information before making any changes to your coverage. **Note:** If you join a Medicare drug plan, you, your spouse, or your dependents may lose your employer or union health coverage.

COBRA—This is a federal law that may allow you to temporarily keep employer or union health coverage after the employment ends or after you lose coverage as a dependent of the covered employee. As explained on pages 26–27, there may be reasons why you should take Part B instead of, or in addition to, COBRA coverage. However, if you take COBRA and it includes creditable prescription drug coverage, you'll have a Special Enrollment Period to join a Medicare drug plan without paying a penalty when the COBRA coverage ends. Talk with your State Health Insurance Assistance Program (SHIP) to see if COBRA is a good choice for you. See pages 141–144 for the phone number.

Medicare Supplement Insurance (Medigap) policy with prescription drug coverage—You may choose to join a Medicare drug plan because most Medigap drug coverage isn't creditable, and you may pay more if you join a drug plan later. See pages 104–105. Medigap policies can no longer be sold with prescription drug coverage, but if you have drug coverage under a current Medigap policy, you can keep it. If you join a Medicare drug plan, tell your Medigap insurance company so they can remove the prescription drug coverage under your Medigap policy and adjust your premiums. Call your Medigap insurance company for more information.

Note: Keep any creditable prescription drug coverage information you get from your plan. You may need it if you decide to join a Medicare drug plan later. Don't send creditable coverage letters or certificates to Medicare.

How does other government insurance work with Part D?

These types of insurance are all considered creditable prescription drug coverage, and in most cases it will be to your advantage to keep this coverage if you have it.

Federal Employee Health Benefits (FEHB) Program—This is health coverage for current and retired federal employees and covered family members. FEHB plans usually include prescription drug coverage, so you don't need to join a Medicare drug plan. However, if you decide to join a Medicare drug plan, you can keep your FEHB plan, and in most cases the Medicare plan will pay first. For more information for retirees, visit opm.gov/healthcare-insurance/healthcare or contact the Office of Personnel Management at 1-888-767-6738. TTY users should call 1-800-878-5707. If you're an active federal employee, you should contact your Benefits Officer. Visit apps.opm.gov/abo for a list of Benefits Officers. You can also call your plan if you have questions.

How does other government insurance work with Part D? (continued)

Veterans' benefits—This is health coverage for veterans and people who have served in the U.S. military. You may be able to get prescription drug coverage through the U.S. Department of Veterans Affairs (VA) program. You may join a Medicare drug plan, but if you do, you can't use both types of coverage for the same prescription at the same time. For more information, visit va.gov, or call the VA at 1-800-827-1000. TTY users should call 1-800-829-4833.

TRICARE (military health benefits)—This is a health care plan for active-duty service members, military retirees, and their families. **Most people with TRICARE who are entitled to Part A must have Part B to keep TRICARE prescription drug benefits.** If you have TRICARE, you don't need to join a Medicare Prescription Drug Plan. However, if you do, your Medicare drug plan pays first, and TRICARE pays second.

If you join a Medicare Advantage Plan (like an HMO or PPO) with prescription drug coverage, your Medicare Advantage Plan and TRICARE may coordinate their benefits if your Medicare Advantage Plan network pharmacy is also a TRICARE network pharmacy. Otherwise, you can file your own claim to get paid back for your out-of-pocket expenses. For more information, visit tricare.mil, or call the TRICARE Pharmacy Program at 1-877-363-1303. TTY users should call 1-877-540-6261.

Indian Health Services (IHS)—The IHS is the primary health care provider to the American Indian/Alaska Native (AI/AN) Medicare population. The Indian health care system, consisting of tribal, urban, and federally operated IHS health programs, delivers a spectrum of clinical and preventive health services through a network of hospitals, clinics, and other entities. Many Indian health facilities participate in the Medicare prescription drug program. If you get prescription drugs through an Indian health facility, you'll continue to get drugs at no cost to you, and your coverage won't be interrupted. Joining a Medicare drug plan may help your Indian health facility because the drug plan pays the Indian health facility for the cost of your prescriptions. Talk to your local Indian health benefits coordinator who can help you choose a plan that meets your needs and tell you how Medicare works with the Indian health care system.

Note: If you're getting care through an IHS or tribal health facility or program without being charged, you can continue to do so for some or all of your care. Getting Medicare doesn't affect your ability to get services through the IHS and tribal health facilities.

Section 8—

Get Help Paying Your Health & Prescription Drug Costs

What if I need help paying my Medicare prescription drug costs?

If you have limited income and resources, you may qualify for help to pay for some health care and prescription drug costs.

Note: Extra Help isn't available in Puerto Rico, the U.S. Virgin Islands, Guam, the Northern Mariana Islands, and American Samoa. See page 118 for information about programs that are available in those areas.

Extra Help is a Medicare program to help people with limited income and resources pay Medicare prescription drug costs. You may qualify for Extra Help if your yearly income and resources are below these limits in 2014:

- Single person—income less than $17,505 and resources less than $13,440 per year
- Married person living with a spouse and no other dependents—income less than $23,595 and resources less than $26,860 per year

These amounts may change in 2015. You may qualify even if you have a higher income (like if you still work, live in Alaska or Hawaii, or have dependents living with you). Resources include money in a checking or savings account, stocks, bonds, mutual funds, and Individual Retirement Accounts (IRAs). Resources **don't** include your home, car, household items, burial plot, up to $1,500 for burial expenses (per person), or life insurance policies.

Definitions of blue words are on pages 145–148.

If you qualify for Extra Help and join a Medicare drug plan, you'll:
- Get help paying your Medicare drug plan's monthly premium, yearly deductible, coinsurance, and copayments.
- Have no coverage gap.
- Have no late enrollment penalty.
- Have the chance to switch plans at any time. Any change you make will take effect the first day of the following month.

You automatically qualify for Extra Help if you have Medicare and meet any of these conditions:
- You have full Medicaid coverage.
- You get help from your state Medicaid program paying your Part B premiums (in a Medicare Savings Program). See pages 115–116.
- You get Supplemental Security Income (SSI) benefits.

To let you know you automatically qualify for Extra Help, Medicare will mail you a purple letter that you should keep for your records. You don't need to apply for Extra Help if you get this letter.
- If you aren't already in a Medicare drug plan, you must join one to use this Extra Help.
- If you don't join a Medicare drug plan, Medicare may enroll you in one so that you'll be able to use the Extra Help. If Medicare enrolls you in a plan, you'll get a yellow or green letter letting you know when your coverage begins.
- Different plans cover different drugs. Check to see if the plan you're enrolled in covers the drugs you use and if you can go to the pharmacies you want. Visit Medicare.gov/find-a-plan, or call 1-800-MEDICARE (1-800-633-4227) to compare with other plans in your area. TTY users should call 1-877-486-2048.
- If you're getting Extra Help, you can switch to another Medicare drug plan anytime. Your new coverage will be effective the first day of the next month.
- If you have Medicaid and live in certain institutions (like a nursing home) or get home- and community-based services, you pay nothing for your covered prescription drugs.

Definitions of blue words are on pages 145–148.

If you don't want to join a Medicare drug plan (for example, because you want only your employer or union coverage), call the plan listed in your letter, or call 1-800-MEDICARE (1-800-633-4227). TTY users should call 1-877-486-2048. Tell them you don't want to be in a Medicare drug plan (you want to "opt out"). If you continue to qualify for Extra Help or if your employer or union coverage is creditable prescription drug coverage, you won't have to pay a penalty if you join later.

Important! If you have employer or union coverage and you join a Medicare drug plan, you may lose your employer or union coverage even if you qualify for Extra Help. Call your employer's benefits administrator before you join a Medicare drug plan.

If you didn't automatically qualify for Extra Help, you can apply at anytime:

- Visit socialsecurity.gov/i1020 to apply online.
- Call Social Security at 1-800-772-1213 to apply for Extra Help by phone or to get a paper application. TTY users should call 1-800-325-0778.
- Visit your State Medical Assistance (Medicaid) office. Visit Medicare.gov/contacts, or call 1-800-MEDICARE to get the phone number.

Note: With your consent, Social Security will forward information to the Medicaid office in your state to start an application for a Medicare Savings Program. See pages 115–116.

Drug costs in 2015 for most people who qualify will be no more than $2.65 for each generic drug and $6.60 for each brand-name drug. Look on the Extra Help letters you get, or contact your plan to find out your exact costs.

To get answers to your questions about Extra Help and help choosing a drug plan, call your State Health Insurance Assistance Program (SHIP). See pages 141–144 for the phone number. You can also call 1-800-MEDICARE.

Paying the right amount

Medicare gets information from your state or Social Security that tells whether you qualify for Extra Help. If Medicare doesn't have the right information, you may be paying the wrong amount for your prescription drug coverage.

If you automatically qualify for Extra Help, you can show your drug plan the colored letter you got from Medicare as proof that you qualify. If you applied for Extra Help, you can show your "Notice of Award" from Social Security as proof that you qualify.

You can also give your plan or pharmacy any of the documents listed in the chart below (also called "Best Available Evidence") as proof that you qualify for Extra Help. **Your plan must accept these documents.** Each item must show that you were eligible for Medicaid during a month after June 2014.

Proof you have Medicaid and live in an institution or get home- and community-based services	Other proof you have Medicaid
■ A bill from the institution (like a nursing home) or a copy of a state document showing Medicaid payment to the institution for at least a month ■ A print-out from your state's Medicaid system showing that you lived in the institution for at least a month ■ A document from your state that shows you have Medicaid and are getting home- and community-based services	■ A copy of your Medicaid card (if you have one) ■ A copy of a state document that shows you have Medicaid ■ A print-out from a state electronic enrollment file or from your state's Medicaid system that shows you have Medicaid ■ Any other document from your state that shows you have Medicaid

Definitions of blue words are on pages 145–148.

If you aren't already enrolled in a Medicare drug plan and paid for prescriptions since you qualified for Extra Help, you may be able to get back part of what you paid. **Keep your receipts**, and call Medicare's Limited Income Newly Eligible Transition (NET) Program at 1-800-783-1307 for more information. TTY users should call 711.

For more information, visit Medicare.gov/publications to view the fact sheet "If You Get Extra Help, Make Sure You're Paying the Right Amount." You can also call 1-800-MEDICARE (1-800-633-4227) to find out if a copy can be mailed to you. TTY users should call 1-877-486-2048.

Note: Keep all information you get from Medicare, Social Security, the Railroad Retirement Board (RRB), your Medicare plan, Medicare Supplement (Medigap) Insurer, employer, or union. This may include notices of award or denial, "Annual Notices of Change," notices of creditable prescription drug coverage, or "Medicare Summary Notices." You may need these documents to apply for the programs explained in this section. Also keep copies of all applications you submit.

What if I need help paying my Medicare health care costs?

Medicare Savings Programs

If you have limited income and resources, you may be able to get help from your state to pay your Medicare costs if you meet certain conditions.

There are 4 kinds of Medicare Savings Programs:

1. **Qualified Medicare Beneficiary (QMB) Program**—Helps pay for Part A and/or Part B premiums, deductibles, coinsurance, and copayments.

2. **Specified Low-Income Medicare Beneficiary (SLMB) Program**—Helps pay Part B premiums only.

3. **Qualifying Individual (QI) Program**—Helps pay Part B premiums only. You must apply each year for QI benefits and the applications are granted on a first-come first-served basis.

4. **Qualified Disabled and Working Individuals (QDWI) Program**—Helps pay Part A premiums only. You may qualify for this program if you have a disability and are working.

Important! The names of these programs and how they work may vary by state. Medicare Savings Programs aren't available in Puerto Rico and the U.S. Virgin Islands.

How do I qualify?

In most cases, to qualify for a Medicare Savings Program, you must have:

- Part A
- Monthly income less than $1,333 and resources less than $7,160—single person
- Monthly income less than $1,790 and resources less than $10,750—married and living together

Note: The amounts above are for 2014 and may change each year. Many states figure your income and resources differently, so you may qualify in your state even if your income or resources are higher than the amounts listed above. If you have income from working, you may qualify for benefits even if your income is higher than the limits above. **Resources** include money in a checking or savings account, stocks, bonds, mutual funds, and Individual Retirement Accounts (IRAs). Resources **don't** include your home, car, burial plot, burial expenses up to your state's limit, furniture, or other household items. Some states don't have any limits on resources.

For more information

- Call or visit your State Medical Assistance (Medicaid) office, and ask for information on Medicare Savings Programs. To get the phone number for your state, visit Medicare.gov/contacts. You can also call 1-800-MEDICARE (1-800-633-4227), and say "Medicaid." TTY users should call 1-877-486-2048.
- Contact your State Health Insurance Assistance Program (SHIP). See pages 141–144 for the phone number.

Medicaid

Medicaid is a joint federal and state program that helps pay medical costs if you have limited income and resources and meet other requirements. Some people qualify for both Medicare and Medicaid and are called "**dual eligibles.**"

What does Medicaid cover?

- If you have Medicare and full Medicaid coverage, most of your health care costs are covered. You can get your Medicare coverage through Original Medicare or a Medicare Advantage Plan (like an HMO or PPO).
- If you have Medicare and full Medicaid coverage, Medicare covers your Part D prescription drugs. Medicaid may still cover some drugs and other care that Medicare doesn't cover.

Definitions of blue words are on pages 145–148.

- People with Medicaid may get coverage for services that Medicare may not or may partially cover, like nursing home care, personal care, and home- and community-based services.

How do I qualify?

- Medicaid programs vary from state to state. They may also have different names, like "Medical Assistance" or "Medi-Cal."
- Each state has different income and resource requirements.
- Many states have expanded their Medicaid programs to cover more people. Even if you were told you didn't qualify for Medicaid in the past, you may qualify under the new rules.
- In some states, you may need to be enrolled in Medicare, if eligible, to get Medicaid.
- Call your State Medical Assistance (Medicaid) office for more information and to see if you qualify. Visit Medicare.gov/contacts, or call 1-800-MEDICARE (1-800-633-4227) and say "Medicaid" to get the phone number. TTY users should call 1-877-486-2048.

Demonstration plans for people who have both Medicare and Medicaid

Medicare is working with several states and health plans to create demonstration plans for certain people who have both Medicare and Medicaid, called Medicare-Medicaid Plans. These plans include all your Medicare and Medicaid benefits, and prescription drug coverage. They're designed to help better coordinate your benefits. If you're interested in joining a Medicare-Medicaid Plan, visit Medicare.gov/find-a-plan to see if one is available in your area and if you qualify. Call your State Medical Assistance (Medicaid) office for more information. Visit Medicare.gov/contacts, or call 1-800-MEDICARE and say "Medicaid" to get the phone number.

State Pharmacy Assistance Programs (SPAPs)

Many states have SPAPs that help certain people pay for prescription drugs based on financial need, age, or medical condition. Each SPAP makes its own rules on how to provide drug coverage to its members. To find out if there's an SPAP in your state and how it works, call your State Health Insurance Assistance Program (SHIP). See pages 141–144 for the phone number.

Pharmaceutical Assistance Programs (also called Patient Assistance Programs)

Many major drug manufacturers offer assistance programs for people with Medicare drug coverage who meet certain requirements. Visit Medicare.gov/pharmaceutical-assistance-program, to learn more about Pharmaceutical Assistance Programs.

Programs of All-inclusive Care for the Elderly (PACE)

PACE is a Medicare and Medicaid program offered in many states that allows people who need a nursing home-level of care to remain in the community. See page 89 for more information.

Supplemental Security Income (SSI) benefits

SSI is a cash benefit paid by Social Security to people with limited income and resources who are disabled, blind, or 65 or older. SSI benefits help people meet basic needs for food, clothing, and shelter. SSI benefits aren't the same as Social Security benefits.

You can visit benefits.gov/ssa, and use the "Benefit Eligibility Screening Tool" to find out if you're eligible for SSI or other benefits. Call Social Security at 1-800-772-1213 or contact your local Social Security office for more information. TTY users should call 1-800-325-0778.

Note: People who live in Puerto Rico, the U.S. Virgin Islands, Guam, or American Samoa can't get SSI.

Programs for people who live in the U.S. territories

There are programs in Puerto Rico, the U.S. Virgin Islands, Guam, the Northern Mariana Islands, and American Samoa to help people with limited income and resources pay their Medicare costs. Programs vary in these areas. Call your local Medical Assistance (Medicaid) office to learn more, or call 1-800-MEDICARE (1-800-633-4227) and say "Medicaid" for more information. TTY users should call 1-877-486-2048.

Definitions of blue words are on pages 145–148.

Section 9—

Know Your Rights & Protect Yourself from Fraud

What are my Medicare rights?

No matter how you get your Medicare, you have certain rights and protections. All people with Medicare have the right to:

- Be treated with dignity and respect at all times
- Be protected from discrimination
- Have their personal and health information kept private
- Get information in a way they understand from Medicare, health care providers, and Medicare contractors
- Have questions about Medicare answered
- Have access to doctors, other health care providers, specialists, and hospitals
- Learn about their treatment choices in clear language that they can understand, and participate in treatment decisions
- Get emergency care when and where they need it
- Get a decision about health care payment, coverage of services, or prescription drug coverage
- Request a review (appeal) of certain decisions about health care payment, coverage of services, or prescription drug coverage
- File complaints (sometimes called "grievances"), including complaints about the quality of their care

What if my plan stops participating in Medicare?

Medicare health and prescription drug plans can decide not to participate in Medicare for the coming year. Plans that choose to leave Medicare entirely or in certain areas are "non-renewing." In these cases, your coverage under the plan will end after December 31. The plan will send you a letter about your options before Open Enrollment. You can choose another plan during Medicare Open Enrollment between October 15–December 7. Your coverage will begin January 1. If your plan is non-renewing for the next year, you'll also have a special right to join another Medicare plan until February 28, 2015.

If you want to continue to have Medicare prescription drug coverage (Part D) or a Medicare Advantage Plan (like an HMO or PPO), without any interruption in coverage, you'll need to join a new plan by December 31. If you **don't** join a new Medicare Advantage Plan by December 31, you'll continue to have Medicare coverage through Original Medicare on January 1, but if you don't join a Medicare drug plan by that date, you won't have Medicare drug coverage.

- Generally, if you're in a Medicare health plan, you'll automatically return to Original Medicare if you don't choose to join another Medicare health plan. You'll also have the right to buy certain Medigap policies within 63 days after your plan coverage ends. If you return to Original Medicare, you can also join a Medicare Prescription Drug Plan.
- If you're in a Medicare drug plan, you'll have the right to join another Medicare drug plan or a Medicare health plan with drug coverage. If you don't join a new plan, you won't have Medicare drug coverage.

What's an appeal?

An appeal is the action you can take if you disagree with a coverage or payment decision by Medicare or your Medicare plan. For example, you can appeal if Medicare or your plan denies:

- A request for a health care service, supply, item, or prescription drug that you think you should be able to get.
- A request for payment of a health care service, supply, item, or prescription drug you already got.
- A request to change the amount you must pay for a health care service, supply, item, or prescription drug.

Definitions of blue words are on pages 145–148.

You can also appeal if Medicare or your plan stops providing or paying for all or part of a health care service, supply, item, or prescription drug you think you still need.

If you decide to file an appeal, you can ask your doctor, supplier, or other health care provider for any information that may help your case. Keep a copy of everything you send to Medicare or your plan as part of your appeal.

How do I file an appeal?

How you file an appeal depends on the type of Medicare coverage you have:

If you have Original Medicare

1. Get the "Medicare Summary Notice" (MSN) that shows the item or service you're appealing. Your MSN is the notice you get every 3 months that lists all the services billed to Medicare and tells you if Medicare paid for the services. See pages 69–70.

2. Circle the item(s) you disagree with on the MSN, and write an explanation of why you disagree with the decision on the MSN or on a separate piece of paper and attach it to the MSN.

3. Include your name, phone number, and Medicare number on the MSN, and sign it. Keep a copy for your records.

4. Send the MSN, or a copy, to the company that handles bills for Medicare listed on the MSN. You can include any other additional information you have about your appeal. Or you can use CMS Form 20027, and file it with the Medicare Administrative Contractor at the address listed on the MSN. To view or print this form, visit cms.gov/cmsforms/downloads/cms20027.pdf, or call 1-800-MEDICARE (1-800-633-4227) to have a copy mailed to you. TTY users should call 1-877-486-2048.

5. You must file the appeal within 120 days of the date you get the MSN in the mail.

You'll generally get a decision from the Medicare Administrative Contractor within 60 days after they get your request. If Medicare will cover the item(s) or service(s), it will be listed on your next MSN.

If you have a Medicare health plan

Learn how to file an appeal by looking at the materials your plan sends you, calling your plan, or visiting Medicare.gov/appeals.

In some cases, you can file a fast appeal. See materials from your plan and page 123.

If you have a Medicare Prescription Drug Plan

You have the right to do all of these (even before you buy a certain drug):

- Get a written explanation (called a "coverage determination") from your Medicare drug plan. A coverage determination is the first decision made by your Medicare drug plan (not the pharmacy) about your benefits, including whether a certain drug is covered, whether you've met the requirements to get a requested drug, how much you pay for a drug, and whether to make an exception to a plan rule when you request it.

- Ask for an exception if you or your prescriber (your doctor or other health care provider who's legally allowed to write prescriptions) believes you need a drug that isn't on your plan's formulary.

- Ask for an exception if you or your prescriber believes that a coverage rule (like prior authorization) should be waived.

- Ask for an exception if you think you should pay less for a higher tier (more expensive) drug because you or your prescriber believes you can't take any of the lower tier (less expensive) drugs for the same condition.

How do I ask for a coverage determination?

You or your prescriber must contact your plan to ask for a coverage determination or an exception. If your network pharmacy can't fill a prescription, the pharmacist will give you a notice that explains how to contact your Medicare drug plan so you can make your request. If the pharmacist doesn't give you this notice, ask for a copy.

Definitions of blue words are on pages 145–148.

You or your prescriber may make a standard request by phone or in writing, if you're asking for prescription drug benefits you haven't gotten yet. If you're asking to get paid back for prescription drugs you already bought, your plan can require you or your prescriber to make the standard request in writing.

You or your prescriber can call or write your plan for an expedited (fast) request. Your request will be expedited if you haven't gotten the prescription and your plan determines, or your prescriber tells your plan, that your life or health may be at risk by waiting.

Important!

If you're requesting an exception, your prescriber must provide a statement explaining the medical reason why the exception should be approved.

What are my rights if I think my services are ending too soon?

If you're getting Medicare services from a hospital, skilled nursing facility, home health agency, comprehensive outpatient rehabilitation facility, or hospice, and you think your Medicare-covered services are ending too soon, you can ask for a fast appeal. Your provider will give you a notice before your services end that will tell you how to ask for a fast appeal. The notice might call it an "expedited determination." You should read this notice carefully. If you don't get this notice, ask your provider for it.

With a fast appeal, an independent reviewer, called a Beneficiary and Family Centered Care Quality Improvement Organization (BFCC-QIO), will decide if your services should continue.

- It's important to call your BFCC-QIO to request a fast appeal no later than the time shown on the notice you get from your provider. Use the phone number for your BFCC-QIO listed on your notice to request your appeal.
- Ask your doctor or other health care provider to submit any information to the BFCC-QIO that may help your case.
- If you miss the deadline, you may still have appeal rights:
    —If you have Original Medicare, call your BFCC-QIO.
    —If you're in a Medicare health plan, call your plan.

How can I get help filing an appeal?

For more information about the different levels of appeals, visit Medicare.gov/appeals. You can also get help filing an appeal from your State Health Insurance Assistance Program (SHIP). See pages 141–144 for the phone number.

What's an "Advance Beneficiary Notice of Noncoverage" (ABN)?

If you have Original Medicare, your doctor, other health care provider, or supplier may give you a notice called an "Advance Beneficiary Notice of Noncoverage" (ABN). This notice says Medicare probably (or certainly) won't pay for some services in certain situations.

What happens if I get an ABN?

- You'll be asked to choose whether to get the items or services listed on the ABN.
- If you choose to get the items or services listed on the ABN, you're agreeing to pay if Medicare doesn't.
- You'll be asked to sign the ABN to say that you've read and understood it.
- Doctors, other health care providers, and suppliers don't have to (but still may) give you an ABN for services that Medicare never covers. See page 62.
- An ABN isn't an official denial of coverage by Medicare. You could choose to get the items listed on the ABN and still ask your health care provider or supplier to submit the claim to Medicare or another insurer. If Medicare denies payment, you can still file an appeal. However, you'll have to pay for the items or services if Medicare determines that the items or services aren't covered (and no other insurer is responsible for payment).

Can I get an ABN for other reasons?

- You may get a "Skilled Nursing Facility ABN" when the facility believes Medicare will no longer cover your stay or other items and services.
- You may get an ABN if you're getting equipment or supplies that are in the DMEPOS Competitive Bidding Program and the supplier isn't a contract supplier.

Definitions of blue words are on pages 145–148.

What if I didn't get an ABN?

If your provider was required to give you an ABN but didn't, in most cases your provider must pay you back what you paid for the item or service.

Where can I get more information about appeals and ABNs?

- Visit Medicare.gov/appeals.
- Visit Medicare.gov/publications to view the booklet "Medicare Appeals." You can also call 1-800-MEDICARE (1-800-633-4227) to find out if a copy can be mailed to you. TTY users should call 1-877-486-2048.
- If you're in a Medicare plan, call your plan to find out if a service or item will be covered.

How does Medicare use my personal information?

Medicare protects the privacy of your health information. The next 2 pages describe how your information may be used and given out by law and explain how you can get this information.

Notice of Privacy Practices for Original Medicare

This notice describes how medical information about you may be used and disclosed and how you can get access to this information. Please review it carefully.

By law, Medicare is required to protect the privacy of your personal medical information. Medicare is also required to give you this notice to tell you how Medicare may use and give out ("disclose") your personal medical information held by Medicare.

Medicare must use and give out your personal medical information to provide information:

- To you, someone you name ("designate"), or someone who has the legal right to act for you (your personal representative)
- To the Secretary of the Department of Health and Human Services, if necessary, to make sure your privacy is protected
- Where required by law

Medicare has the right to use and give out your personal medical information to pay for your health care and to operate the Medicare Program. Examples include:

- Companies that pay bills for Medicare use your personal medical information to pay or deny your claims, to collect your premiums, to share your payment information with your other insurer(s), or to prepare your "Medicare Summary Notice."
- Medicare may use your personal medical information to make sure you and other people with Medicare get quality health care, to provide customer service to you, to resolve any complaints you have, or to contact you about research studies.

Medicare may use or give out your personal medical information for these purposes under limited circumstances:

- Where allowed by federal law to state and other federal agencies that need Medicare data for their program operations (like to make sure Medicare is making proper payments or to coordinate benefits between programs)
- To your health care providers so they know what other treatments you've gotten and to coordinate your care (for example, for programs to ensure the delivery of quality health care)
- For public health activities (like reporting disease outbreaks)
- For government health care oversight activities (like fraud and abuse investigations)
- For judicial and administrative proceedings (like in response to a court order)
- For law enforcement purposes (like providing limited information to locate a missing person)
- For research studies, including surveys, that meet all privacy law requirements (like research related to the prevention of disease or disability)
- To avoid a serious and imminent threat to health or safety
- To contact you about new or changed coverage under Medicare

- To create a collection of information that can no longer be traced back to you

By law, Medicare must have your written permission (an "authorization") to use or give out your personal medical information for any purpose that isn't set out in this notice. Medicare will not sell or market your personal medical information without your written permission. You may take back ("revoke") your written permission anytime, except to the extent that Medicare has already acted based on your permission.

By law, you have the right to:

- See and get a copy of your personal medical information held by Medicare.

- Have your personal medical information amended if you believe that it is wrong or if information is missing, and Medicare agrees. If Medicare disagrees, you may have a statement of your disagreement added to your personal medical information.

- Get a listing of those getting your personal medical information from Medicare. The listing won't cover your personal medical information that was given to you or your personal representative, that was given out to pay for your health care or for Medicare operations, or that was given out for law enforcement purposes if it would likely get in the way of these purposes.

- Ask Medicare to communicate with you in a different manner or at a different place (for example, by sending materials to a P.O. Box instead of your home address).

- Ask Medicare to limit how your personal medical information is used and given out to pay your claims and run the Medicare Program. Please note that Medicare may not be able to agree to your request.

- Be told about any breach of your personal medical information.

- Get a separate paper copy of this notice.

Visit Medicare.gov for more information on:

- Exercising your rights set out in this notice.

- Filing a complaint, if you believe Original Medicare has violated these privacy rights. Filing a complaint won't affect your coverage under Medicare.

You can also call 1-800-MEDICARE (1-800-633-4227) to get this information. Ask to speak to a customer service representative about Medicare's privacy notice. TTY users should call 1-877-486-2048.

You may file a complaint with the Secretary of the Department of Health and Human Services. Call the Office for Civil Rights at 1-800-368-1019. TTY users should call 1-800-537-7697. You can also visit hhs.gov/ocr/privacy.

By law, Medicare is required to follow the terms in this privacy notice. Medicare has the right to change the way your personal medical information is used and given out. If Medicare makes any changes to the way your personal medical information is used and given out, you'll get a new notice by mail within 60 days of the change.

The Notice of Privacy Practices for Original Medicare is effective September 23, 2013.

How can I protect myself from identity theft?

Identity theft happens when someone uses your personal information without your consent to commit fraud or other crimes. Personal information includes things like your name and your Social Security, Medicare, credit card, or bank account numbers. Guard your cards and protect your Medicare and Social Security numbers. **Keep this information safe.**

Only give personal information, like your Medicare number, to doctors, other health care providers, and plans approved by Medicare; any insurer who pays benefits on your behalf; and to trusted people in the community who work with Medicare, like your State Health Insurance Assistance Program (SHIP) or Social Security. Call 1-800-MEDICARE (1-800-633-4227) if you aren't sure if a provider is approved by Medicare. TTY users should call 1-877-486-2048.

If you suspect identity theft, or feel like you gave your personal information to someone you shouldn't have, call your local police department and the Federal Trade Commission's ID Theft Hotline at 1-877-438-4338. TTY users should call 1-866-653-4261. Visit ftc.gov/idtheft to learn more about identity theft.

How can I protect myself and Medicare from fraud?

Most doctors, pharmacists, plans, and other health care providers who work with Medicare are honest. Unfortunately, there may be some who are dishonest. One common form of Medicare fraud is when Medicare is billed for services you never got. Medicare fraud costs everyone a lot of money each year.

Definitions of blue words are on pages 145–148.

Check your statements for mistakes

When you get health care services, record the dates on a calendar and save the receipts and statements you get from providers to

check for mistakes. If you think you see an error or are billed for services you didn't get, do these to find out what was billed:

- Check your "Medicare Summary Notice" (MSN) if you have Original Medicare to see if the service was billed to Medicare. If you're in a Medicare plan, check the statements you get from your plan.

- If you know the health care provider or supplier, call and ask for an itemized statement. They should give this to you within 30 days.

- Visit MyMedicare.gov to view your Medicare claims if you have Original Medicare. Your claims are generally available online within 24 hours after processing. You can also download your claims information by using Medicare's Blue Button. See page 135. The sooner you see and report errors, the sooner we can stop fraud. You can also call 1-800-MEDICARE (1-800-633-4227). TTY users should call 1-877-486-2048.

If you've contacted the provider and you suspect that Medicare is being charged for a service or supply that you didn't get, or you don't know the provider on the claim, call 1-800-MEDICARE.

For more information on protecting yourself from Medicare fraud and tips for spotting and reporting fraud, visit stopmedicarefraud.gov, or contact your local Senior Medicare Patrol (SMP) Program. See page 130.

You can also visit oig.hhs.gov or call the fraud hotline of the Department of Health and Human Services Office of the Inspector General at 1-800-HHS-TIPS (1-800-447-8477). TTY users should call 1-800-377-4950.

Plans must follow rules

Medicare plans must follow certain rules when marketing their plans and getting your enrollment information. They can't ask you for credit card or banking information over the phone or via email, unless you're already a member of that plan. Medicare plans can't enroll you into a plan over the phone unless you call them and ask to enroll, or you've given them permission to contact you.

Important! ▶ **Call 1-800-MEDICARE (1-800-633-4227) to report any plans that:**

- Ask for your personal information over the phone or email
- Call to enroll you in a plan
- Use false information to mislead you

You can also call the Medicare Drug Integrity Contractor (MEDIC) at 1-877-7SAFERX (1-877-772-3379). The MEDIC helps prevent inappropriate activity and fights fraud, waste, and abuse in Medicare Advantage (Part C) and Medicare Prescription Drug (Part D) Programs.

For more information on the rules that Medicare plans must follow, visit Medicare.gov/publications to view the booklet "Protecting Medicare and You from Fraud." You can also call 1-800-MEDICARE (1-800-633-4227) to find out if a copy can be mailed to you. TTY users should call 1-877-486-2048.

What's the Senior Medicare Patrol (SMP) Program?

The SMP Program educates and empowers people with Medicare to take an active role in detecting and preventing health care fraud and abuse. The SMP Program not only protects people with Medicare, it also helps preserve Medicare. There's an SMP Program in every state, the District of Columbia, Guam, the U.S. Virgin Islands, and Puerto Rico. Contact your local SMP Program to get personalized counseling, find out about community events in your area, or volunteer. For more information or to find your local SMP Program, visit smpresource.org, or call 1-877-808-2468. You can also call 1-800-MEDICARE.

Fighting fraud can pay

Definitions of blue words are on pages 145–148.

You may get a reward if you help us fight fraud and meet certain conditions. For more information, visit stopmedicarefraud.gov or Medicare.gov, or call 1-800-MEDICARE.

Investigating fraud takes time

Every tip counts. Medicare takes all reports of suspected fraud seriously. When you report fraud, you may not hear of an outcome right away. It takes time to investigate your report and build a case — but rest assured that your information is helping us protect Medicare.

Is my right to my own health information protected?

In most cases, you have the right to request and receive copies of your personal health records in an electronic or paper format from any health care provider. Your health information rights include the right to:

- Access your health information in a paper or electronic format
- Know who has seen your health information
- Correct or amend your health information
- Receive a notice of privacy practices (a privacy policy)
- File a complaint

For more information, or if you think your rights have been violated, visit hhs.gov/ocr or call the Department of Health and Human Services, Office for Civil Rights at 1-800-368-1019. TTY users should call 1-800-537-7697.

What's the Medicare Beneficiary Ombudsman?

An "ombudsman" is a person who reviews complaints and helps resolve them. The Medicare Beneficiary Ombudsman makes sure you have information about:

- Your Medicare coverage
- Making good health care decisions
- Your Medicare rights and protections
- Getting issues resolved

The Ombudsman reviews the concerns raised by people with Medicare through 1-800-MEDICARE and through your State Health Insurance Assistance Program (SHIP).

Visit Medicare.gov for information on inquiries and complaints, activities of the Ombudsman, and what people with Medicare need to know.

What are advance directives?

Advance directives are legal documents that allow you to put in writing what kind of health care you would want or name someone who can speak for you if you were too ill to speak for yourself.

These legal documents help ensure your wishes are followed, but it's important to talk to your family, friends, and health care providers about your wishes. You should also make sure that your family, friends, and health care providers have copies of your legal documents. It's better to think about these important decisions and have plans in place before you're ill or a crisis strikes.

Advance directives most often include:

- **A health care proxy** (sometimes called a "durable power of attorney for health care"). This is used to name the person you want to make health care decisions for you if you aren't able to make them yourself.
- **A living will.** This is another way to make sure your voice is heard. It states which medical treatment you would accept or refuse if your life is threatened.
- **After-death wishes.** These may include choices like organ and tissue donation.

Each state has its own laws for creating advance directives. Some states may allow you to combine your advance directives in one document.

What if I already have an advance directive?

Take time now to review your advance directive to be sure you're still satisfied with your decisions and the person you identify in your health care proxy is still willing and able to carry out your plans. Find out how to cancel or update it in your state if it no longer reflect your wishes.

Definitions of blue words are on pages 145–148.

For more information, contact your health care provider, an attorney, your local Area Agency on Aging, your state health department, or visit Eldercare.gov.

Section 10 —

Get More Information

Where can I get personalized help?

1-800-MEDICARE (1-800-633-4227)

TTY users call 1-877-486-2048

Get information 24 hours a day, including weekends

- Speak clearly, have your Medicare card in front of you, and be ready to provide your Medicare number. This helps reduce the amount of time you may wait to speak to a customer service representative. It also allows us to play messages that may specifically impact your coverage and may help us get you to a representative more quickly.

- To enter your Medicare number, speak the numbers and letter(s) clearly one at a time. Or, enter your Medicare number on the phone keypad. Use the star key to indicate any place there may be a letter. For example, if your Medicare number is 000-00-0000A, you would enter 0-0-0-0-0- 0-0-0-0-*. The voice system will then ask you for that letter.

- Use 1 or 2 words to briefly say what you're calling about.

Tip: You can say "Agent" at any time to talk to a customer service representative.

If you need help in a language other than English or Spanish, let the customer service representative know.

Important! If you want someone to be able to call 1-800-MEDICARE on your behalf, you need to let Medicare know in writing. You can fill out a "Medicare Authorization to Disclose Personal Health Information" form so Medicare can give your personal health

information to someone other than you. You can do this by visiting Medicare.gov/medicareonlineforms or by calling 1-800-MEDICARE (1-800-633-4227) to get a copy of the form. TTY users should call 1-877-486-2048. You may want to do this now in case you become unable to do it later.

People who get benefits from the Railroad Retirement Board (RRB) should call 1-800-833-4455 with questions about Part B services and bills.

Did your household get more than one copy of "Medicare & You?"

If you want to get only one copy in the future, call 1-800-MEDICARE. If you want to get the handbook electronically and not get any future copies in the mail, visit Medicare.gov/gopaperless.

What are State Health Insurance Assistance Programs (SHIPs)?

SHIPs are state programs that get money from the federal government to give local health insurance counseling to people with Medicare. SHIPs aren't connected to any insurance company or health plan. SHIP volunteers work hard to help you with these Medicare questions or concerns:

- Your Medicare rights
- Billing problems
- Complaints about your medical care or treatment
- Plan choices
- How Medicare works with other insurance

Definitions of blue words are on pages 145–148.

See pages 141–144 for the phone number of your local SHIP. If you would like to become a volunteer SHIP counselor, contact the SHIP in your state to learn more.

Where can I find general Medicare information online?

Visit Medicare.gov

- Get detailed information about the Medicare health and prescription drug plans in your area, including what they cost and what services they provide.
- Find doctors or other health care providers and suppliers who participate in Medicare.
- See what Medicare covers, including preventive services.
- Get Medicare appeals information and forms.
- Get information about the quality of care provided by plans, nursing homes, hospitals, home health agencies, and dialysis facilities.
- Look up helpful websites and phone numbers.

Where can I find personalized Medicare information online?

Register at MyMedicare.gov

- Complete your "Initial Enrollment Questionnaire" so your claims can get paid correctly.
- Manage your personal information (like medical conditions, allergies, and implanted devices).
- Sign up to get this handbook electronically. You won't get a printed copy if you choose to get it electronically.
- Manage your personal drug list and pharmacy information.
- Search for, add to, and manage a list of your favorite providers and access quality information about them.
- Track Original Medicare claims and your Part B deductible status.
- View and order copies of your "Medicare Summary Notices."

Get access to your personal health information using Medicare's Blue Button. This feature lets you download 12–36 months of claims information for Part A and Part B and 12 months of claims information for Part D. This information can help you make more informed decisions about your care and can give your health care providers a more complete view of your health history. Visit MyMedicare.gov to use the Blue Button today.

Once you've used the Blue Button, there are a variety of health applications and services to analyze your health information. Visit bluebuttonconnector.healthit.gov to learn more about these useful tools and how to protect your health information once it's in your hands.

How do I compare the quality of plans and providers?

Medicare collects information about the quality and safety of medical care and services given by most Medicare plans and health care providers. Medicare also has information about the experiences of people with the care and services they get.

Compare the quality of care (how well plans and providers work to give you the best care possible) and services given by health and prescription drug plans or health care providers nationwide by visiting Medicare.gov or by calling your State Health Insurance Assistance Program (SHIP). See pages 141–144 for the phone number.

When you, a family member, friend, or SHIP counselor visit Medicare.gov, use these tools:

- Hospital Compare
- Nursing Home Compare
- Home Health Compare
- Dialysis Facility Compare
- Physician Compare
- Medicare Plan Finder

Definitions of blue words are on pages 145–148.

These search tools on Medicare.gov give you a "snapshot" of the quality of care and services some plans and providers give. Medicare Plan Finder and Nursing Home Compare both feature a star rating system to help you compare plans and quality of care measures that are important to you. Find out more about the quality of care and services by:

- Asking what your plan or provider does to ensure and improve the quality of care and services. Each plan and health care provider should have someone you can talk to about quality.

- Asking your doctor or other health care provider what he or she thinks about the quality of care or services the plan or other providers give. You can also talk to your doctor or other health care provider about Medicare's information on quality of care and services.

What's Medicare doing to better coordinate my care?

Medicare continues to look for ways to better coordinate your care and to make sure that you get the best health care possible. Health information technology (also called "Health IT") and improved ways to deliver your care can help manage your health information, improve how you communicate with your health care providers, and improve the quality and coordination of your health care. These tools also reduce paperwork, medical errors, and health care costs.

Here are examples of how your **health care providers** can better coordinate your care:

Electronic Health Records (EHRs)—EHRs are records that your doctor, other health care provider, medical office staff, or a hospital keeps on a computer about your health care or treatments.

- EHRs can help lower the chances of medical errors, eliminate duplicate tests, and may improve your overall quality of care.

- Your doctor's EHR may be able to link to a hospital, lab, pharmacy, or other doctors, so the people who care for you can have a more complete picture of your health. You also have the right to get a copy of your health information for your own personal use and to make sure the information is complete and accurate.

Electronic prescribing—This is an electronic way for your prescribers (your doctor or other health care provider who is legally allowed to write prescriptions) to send your prescriptions directly to your pharmacy. Electronic prescribing can save you money, time, and help keep you safe.

- You don't have to drop off and wait for your prescription. Your prescription may be ready when you arrive.
- Prescribers can check which drugs your insurance covers and may be able to prescribe a drug that costs you less.
- Electronic prescriptions are easier for the pharmacist to read than handwritten prescriptions. This means there's less chance that you'll get the wrong drug or dose.
- Prescribers can be alerted to potential drug interactions, allergies, and other warnings.

Accountable Care Organizations (ACOs)—An ACO is a group of doctors and other health care providers who agree to work together with Medicare to give you more coordinated service and care. ACOs are designed to help your doctors or primary care providers communicate closely with your other health care providers, so they can deliver high-quality care that meets your individual needs and preferences.

If you have Original Medicare and your doctor has decided to participate in an ACO, you'll be notified (either in person or by letter) that your doctor is participating in an ACO.

The notice will also inform you that Medicare may share information about care you received from your doctors and other providers. With this information, the doctors and health care providers in the ACO can have a complete picture of your health and be better able to coordinate your care. Talk with your doctor or call 1-800-MEDICARE (1-800-633-4227) if you have any questions about the information Medicare may share with the ACO in which your doctor participates. TTY users should call 1-877-486-2048.

Your Medicare benefits, services, costs, and protections won't change if your doctor participates in an ACO. You still have the right to visit and receive care from any doctor or hospital that accepts Medicare at any time, the same way you do now.

For more information, visit Medicare.gov/acos.html, or call 1-800-MEDICARE.

Definitions of blue words are on pages 145–148.

Are there other ways to get Medicare information?

Publications

Visit Medicare.gov/publications to view, print, or download copies of booklets, brochures, or fact sheets on different Medicare topics. You can search by keyword (like "rights" or "mental health"), or select "View all publications." If the publication you want has an "Order" button, you can have a printed copy mailed to you. You can also call 1-800-MEDICARE (1-800-633-4227) and say "Publications" to have a printed copy mailed to you. TTY users should call 1-877-486-2048. Alternate formats are available at no cost. See the inside of the back cover for more information about auxiliary aids and services for people with disabilities.

Videos

Visit YouTube.com/cmshhsgov to see videos covering different health care topics on Medicare's YouTube channel.

Blogs

Visit blog.medicare.gov for up-to-date news from our website.

Resources for caregivers

Medicare has resources to help caregivers get the information they need. To find out more:

- Visit Medicare.gov/caregivers to help someone you care for choose a drug plan, compare nursing homes, get help with billing, and more.
- Visit the Eldercare Locator, a public service of the U.S. Administration on Aging, at Eldercare.gov, or call 1-800-677-1116 to find caregiver support services in your area.
- Visit the Patients & Families section of HealthIT.gov for information about online resources and other eHealth tools designed to support caregivers.

Open Payments Program

Sometimes, doctors and hospitals have financial relationships with health care manufacturing companies. These relationships can include money for research activities, gifts, speaking fees, meals, or travel. Open Payments is a federally run program that collects information about these financial relationships and makes it available to you. Soon, Open Payments will create a public, national database that you can use. You'll be able to look up your health care providers, see if they have any of these relationships, and be more informed about how these relationships may impact your health care decisions. We encourage you to discuss these relationships with your health care providers. Visit go.cms.gov/openpayments for more information.

State Health Insurance Assistance Program (SHIPs)

For help with questions about appeals, buying other insurance, choosing a health plan, buying a Medigap policy, and Medicare rights and protections.

This page has been intentionally left blank. The printed version contains phone number information. For the most recent phone number information, please visit Medicare.gov/contacts. Thank you.

This page has been intentionally left blank. The printed version contains phone number information. For the most recent phone number information, please visit Medicare.gov/contacts. Thank you.

This page has been intentionally left blank. The printed version contains phone number information. For the most recent phone number information, please visit Medicare.gov/contacts. Thank you.

This page has been intentionally left blank. The printed version contains phone number information. For the most recent phone number information, please visit Medicare.gov/contacts. Thank you.

Section 11—Definitions

Assignment—An agreement by your doctor, provider, or supplier to be paid directly by Medicare, to accept the payment amount Medicare approves for the service, and not to bill you for any more than the Medicare deductible and coinsurance.

Benefit period—The way that Original Medicare measures your use of hospital and skilled nursing facility (SNF) services. A benefit period begins the day you're admitted as an inpatient in a hospital or SNF. The benefit period ends when you haven't received any inpatient hospital care (or skilled care in a SNF) for 60 days in a row. If you go into a hospital or a SNF after one benefit period has ended, a new benefit period begins. You must pay the inpatient hospital deductible for each benefit period. There's no limit to the number of benefit periods.

Coinsurance—An amount you may be required to pay as your share of the cost for services after you pay any deductibles. Coinsurance is usually a percentage (for example, 20%).

Copayment—An amount you may be required to pay as your share of the cost for a medical service or supply, like a doctor's visit, hospital outpatient visit, or prescription drug. A copayment is usually a set amount, rather than a percentage. For example, you might pay $10 or $20 for a doctor's visit or prescription drug.

Creditable prescription drug coverage—Prescription drug coverage (for example, from an employer or union) that's expected to pay, on average, at least as much as Medicare's standard prescription drug coverage. People who have this kind of coverage when they become eligible for Medicare can generally keep that coverage without paying a penalty if they decide to enroll in Medicare prescription drug coverage later.

Critical access hospital—A small facility that provides outpatient services, as well as inpatient services on a limited basis, to people in rural areas.

Custodial care—Nonskilled personal care, like help with activities of daily living like bathing, dressing, eating, getting in or out of a bed or chair, moving around, and using the bathroom. It may also include the kind of health-related care that most people do themselves, like using eye drops. In most cases, Medicare doesn't pay for custodial care.

Deductible—The amount you must pay for health care or prescriptions before Original Medicare, your Medicare Advantage Plan, your prescription drug plan, or your other insurance begins to pay.

Demonstrations—Special projects, sometimes called "pilot programs" or "research studies," that test improvements in Medicare coverage, payment, and quality of care. They usually only operate for a limited time, for a specific group of people, and in specific areas.

Extra Help—A Medicare program to help people with limited income and resources pay Medicare prescription drug plan costs, like premiums, deductibles, and coinsurance.

Formulary—A list of prescription drugs covered by a prescription drug plan or another insurance plan offering prescription drug benefits. This is also called a drug list.

Inpatient rehabilitation facility—A hospital, or part of a hospital, that provides an intensive rehabilitation program to inpatients.

Institution—For the purposes of this publication, an institution is a facility that provides short-term or long-term care, such as a nursing home, skilled nursing facility (SNF), or rehabilitation hospital. Private residences, like an assisted living facility or group home, aren't considered institutions for this purpose.

Lifetime reserve days—In Original Medicare, these are additional days that Medicare will pay for when you're in a hospital for more than 90 days. You have a total of 60 reserve days that can be used during your lifetime. For each lifetime reserve day, Medicare pays all covered costs except for a daily coinsurance.

Long-term care—Services that include medical and non-medical care provided to people who are unable to perform basic activities of daily living, like dressing or bathing. Long-term supports and services can be provided at home, in the community, in assisted living, or in nursing homes. Individuals may need long-term supports and services at any age. Medicare and most health insurance plans don't pay for long-term care.

Long-term care hospital—Acute care hospitals that provide treatment for patients who stay, on average, more than 25 days. Most patients are transferred from an intensive or critical care unit. Services provided include comprehensive rehabilitation, respiratory therapy, head trauma treatment, and pain management.

Medically necessary—Health care services or supplies needed to prevent, diagnose, or treat an illness, injury, condition, disease, or its symptoms and that meet accepted standards of medicine.

Medicare-approved amount—In Original Medicare, this is the amount a doctor or supplier that accepts assignment can be paid. It may be less than the actual amount a doctor or supplier charges. Medicare pays part of this amount and you're responsible for the difference.

Medicare health plan—A plan offered by a private company that contracts with Medicare to provide Part A and Part B benefits to people with Medicare who enroll in the plan. Medicare health plans include all Medicare Advantage Plans, Medicare Cost Plans, Demonstration/Pilot Programs and Programs of All-inclusive Care for the Elderly (PACE).

Medicare plan—Refers to any way other than Original Medicare that you can get your Medicare health or prescription drug coverage. This term includes all Medicare health plans and Medicare Prescription Drug Plans.

Premium—The periodic payment to Medicare, an insurance company, or a health care plan for health or prescription drug coverage.

Preventive services—Health care to prevent illness or detect illness at an early stage, when treatment is likely to work best (for example, preventive services include Pap tests, flu shots, and screening mammograms).

Primary care doctor—The doctor you see first for most health problems. He or she makes sure you get the care you need to keep you healthy. He or she also may talk with other doctors and health care providers about your care and refer you to them. In many Medicare Advantage Plans, you must see your primary care doctor before you see any other health care provider.

Primary care practitioner—A doctor who has a primary specialty in family medicine, internal medicine, geriatric medicine, or pediatric medicine; or a nurse practitioner, clinical nurse specialist, or physician assistant.

Quality Improvement Organization (QIO)—A group of practicing doctors and other health care experts paid by the federal government to check and improve the care given to people with Medicare.

Referral—A written order from your primary care doctor for you to see a specialist or get certain medical services. In many Health Maintenance Organizations (HMOs), you need to get a referral before you can get medical care from anyone except your primary care doctor. If you don't get a referral first, the plan may not pay for the services.

Service area—A geographic area where a health insurance plan accepts members if it limits membership based on where people live. For plans that limit which doctors and hospitals you may use, it's also generally the area where you can get routine (non-emergency) services. The plan may disenroll you if you move out of the plan's service area.

Skilled nursing facility (SNF) care—Skilled nursing care and rehabilitation services provided on a continuous, daily basis, in a skilled nursing facility.

TTY—A teletypewriter (TTY) is a communication device used by people who are deaf, hard-of-hearing, or have a severe speech impairment. People who don't have a TTY can communicate with a TTY user through a message relay center (MRC). An MRC has TTY operators available to send and interpret TTY messages.

Notes

Part A and Part B costs

The 2015 premium and deductible amounts for Part A and Part B weren't available at the time of printing. To get the most up-to-date information on these costs, visit Medicare.gov/your-medicare-costs or call 1-800-MEDICARE (1-800-633-4227). TTY users should call 1-877-486-2048. Part C and Part D (Medicare health and prescription drug plans) costs for covered services and supplies for the Medicare plans in your area can be found by:

- Visiting Medicare.gov/find-a-plan.
- Contacting the plan.
- Calling 1-800-MEDICARE.
- Calling your State Health Insurance Assistance Program (SHIP). See pages 141–144 for the phone number.

Medicare Advantage Plans (like an HMO or PPO) must cover all Part A and Part B-covered services and supplies. Check your plan's materials for actual amounts.

Definitions of blue words are on pages 145–148.

Medicare cares about what you think. If you have general comments about this handbook, email us at medicareandyou@cms.hhs.gov. We can't respond to every comment, but we'll consider your feedback when writing future handbooks.

Nondiscrimination Notice

Medicare and every company or agency that works with Medicare must obey the law. Accordingly, you can't be treated unfairly because of your race, color, national origin, disability, age, or sex. If you think that you've been discriminated against or treated unfairly for any of these reasons, call the Department of Health and Human Services, Office for Civil Rights at 1-800-368-1019. TTY users should call 1-800-537-7697. You can also visit hhs.gov/ocr for more information about your rights and how to file a complaint.

Auxiliary aids and services for people with disabilities

Medicare is committed to making its programs, benefits, services, facilities, information, and technology accessible to everyone, in accordance with Sections 504 and 508 of the Rehabilitation Act of 1973. Medicare will take appropriate steps to make sure that people with disabilities, including people who are deaf, hard of hearing, blind, or who have low vision or other sensory limitations, have an equal opportunity to participate in its services, activities, programs, and other benefits. Medicare provides various auxiliary aids and services to communicate with people with disabilities, including:

- **Relay service**
  Medicare uses relay services for telephone communication with external TTY users. Medicare accepts and makes calls through a relay service. The relay service number is 1-877-486-2048.

- **Alternate formats**
  Medicare documents, including this handbook, are available in alternate formats, including: large print, Braille, and audio.

**U.S. DEPARTMENT OF
HEALTH AND HUMAN SERVICES**

Centers for Medicare & Medicaid Services
7500 Security Boulevard
Baltimore, Maryland 21244-1850

Official Business
Penalty for Private Use, $300

CMS Product No. 10050
September 2014

National Medicare Handbook

- Also available in Spanish and alternate formats, including Braille, CD, and large print.
- Moving? Visit socialsecurity.gov, or call Social Security at 1-800-772-1213. TTY users should call 1-800-325-0778. If you get RRB benefits, contact the RRB at 1-877-772-5772. TTY users should call 1-312-751-4701.

¿Necesita usted una copia de este manual en Español?
Llame al 1-800-MEDICARE (1-800-633-4227).
Los usuarios de TTY deberán llamar al 1-877-486-2048.

If you need help in a language other than English or Spanish, call 1-800-MEDICARE and say "Agent." Then tell the customer service representative the language you speak, so you can get free interpretation services.

Medicare.gov
1-800-MEDICARE (1-800-633-4227)
TTY 1-877-486-2048

10% recycled paper

Made in the USA
Middletown, DE
12 March 2015